Color Atlas of Ocular Tumors

Library of Congress Cataloging in Publication Data

Bedford, Michael Alison.
    Color Atlas of Ocular Tumors
    Bibliography: p
    Includes Index
    1. Eye – Tumors – Atlases. 1. Title. (DNLM:
1. Eye Neoplasms – Atlases. WW17 B411ca)
RC280. E9B44   616.9′92′84   79–16497
ISBN 0–8151–0627–0

Color Atlas of
Ocular Tumors

Year Book Medical Publishers, Inc
35 East Wacker Drive, Chicago

Acknowledgements

I would like to thank all those eye surgeons, radiotherapists and paediatricians who have referred patients to me over the last fourteen years. Without these many sources it would have been impossible to study such a relatively large number of rare conditions and to produce this Atlas in an attempt to familiarise other clinicians who have not had the good fortune to 'sub-specialise' as I have.

Additional thanks are due to my secretary Wendy Taylor for her tolerance and efficiency.

Contents

Introduction

Many of the tumours that can involve the eye and lids are rare. The relatively infrequent occurrence of these tumours precludes the average eye surgeon from becoming familiar with them at their varying stages of development or in their differential diagnoses.

It is felt, therefore, that there is a need for an essentially clinical, photographic presentation of these cases showing their various manifestations, together with some indication of their management and the side-effects of various forms of therapy. This Atlas is intended to fill that need.

The tumours will be discussed under the following headings: Skin tumours; Conjunctival tumours; Uveal tumours – iris, ciliary body, choroid; Retinal tumours.

Skin tumours

These tumours are the most common that the average eye surgeon will meet but even so the diagnosis is sometimes missed, perhaps because the average clinician is not 'cancer conscious'.

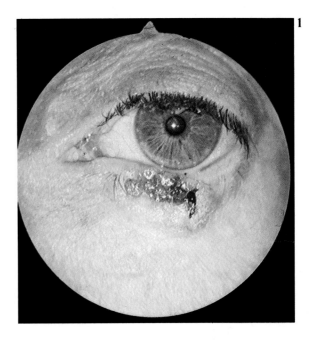

1 The main features of a typical basal cell carcinoma or rodent ulcer. Thus, there is the presence of a slowly growing lesion with a central ulcerated area surrounded by a rolled outer margin with fine blood vessels in it. The lashes involved are missing or distorted. The diagnosis is obvious but *must* be proven by biopsy, or by a scraping by a competent cytologist. The reason for this is that no adequate treatment can be carried out unless the diagnosis is certain (see Figure 2).

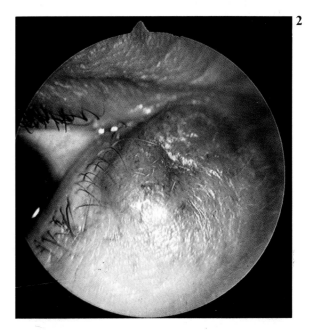

2 A case referred as a 'typical rodent ulcer'. Biopsy showed a 'lymphoma'. The extreme differences in treatment and follow-up of these two diseases need not be stressed.

The series of cases Figures 3–10 were each referred with a diagnosis of 'basal cell carcinoma'.

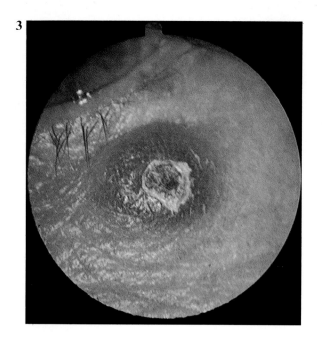

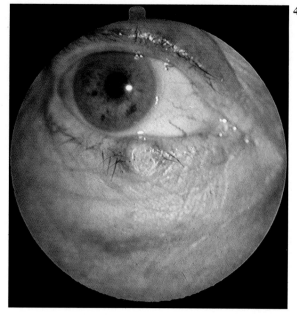

3 A case referred as a basal cell carcinoma. Histological diagnosis showed a sebaceous cyst.

4 A case referred as a basal cell carcinoma. Histological diagnosis showed a keratoacanthoma. Note the central plug of keratin.

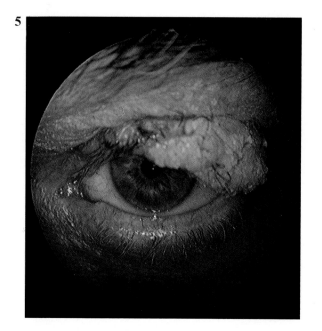

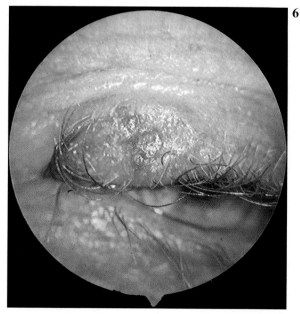

5 A case referred as a basal cell carcinoma. Biopsy in two places showed a keratoacanthoma in one and a squamous cell carcinoma in the other.

6 A case referred as a basal cell carcinoma. Histological diagnosis showed a squamous cell carcinoma.

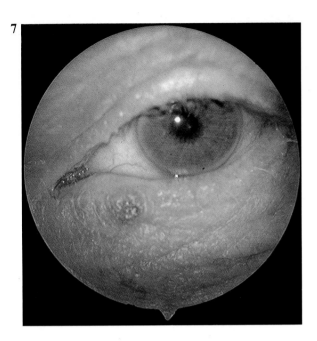

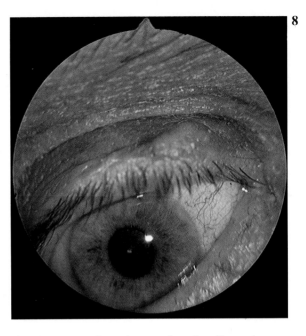

7 A case referred as a basal cell carcinoma. Histological diagnosis showed a senile keratosis.

8 A case referred as a basal cell carcinoma. Histological diagnosis showed a reticulohistio-cytoma.

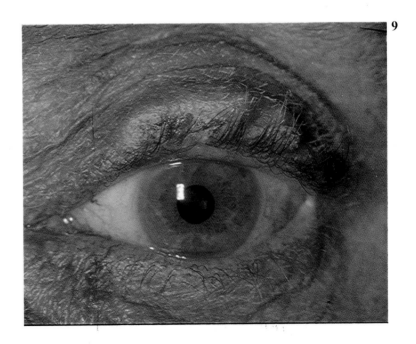

9 A case referred as a basal cell carcinoma. Histology showed a non-specific inflammatory lesion with no evidence of neoplasia.

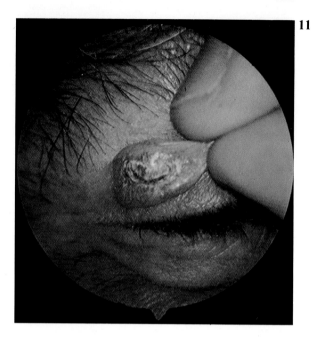

10 A case referred as a basal cell carcinoma. Histology showed a non-specific angiomatous lesion.

11 The lesion is mobile enough, occasionally, with sufficient loose skin surrounding it, to be removed completely as a simple excision biopsy.

Thus, in the management of these cases the precise histological diagnosis is vital before any treatment is undertaken. In every case, a biopsy or a scraping should be undertaken.

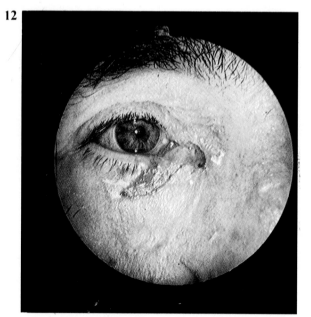

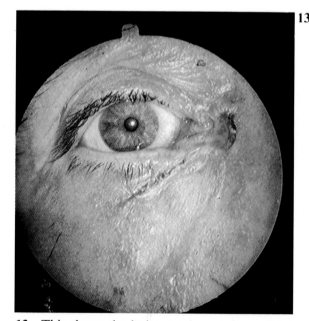

12 In the diagnosis of suspicious lesions near the medial canthus involving the tear passages, there may be a considerable infective element present so that the malignant lesion appears to be more widespread than it is.

13 This shows the lesion as above, after a short course of antibiotics reduced its extent considerably and a biopsy then confirmed the diagnosis of a basal cell carcinoma.

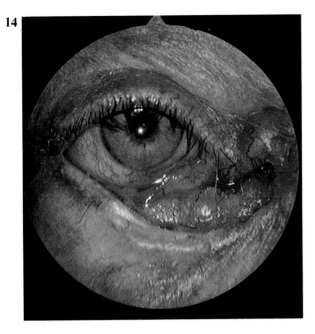

14 At other times there is no infective element, the whole lesion being neoplastic.

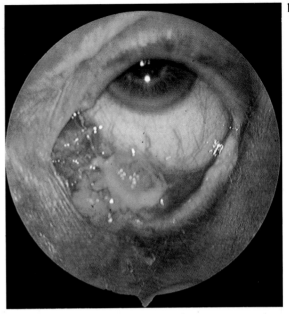

15 Occasionally the lesion proliferates extensively from the skin into the conjunctival sac, so masking the correct diagnosis. A biopsy showed a basal cell carcinoma arising from the skin.

SIDE-EFFECTS OF THERAPY
Gross side-effects should be seen rarely.

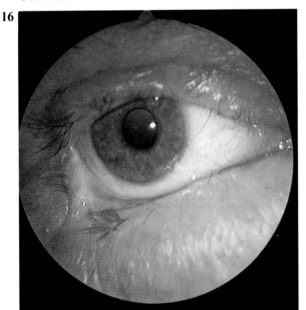

16 Shows the disfiguring appearances of bulky skin flaps following an unnecessary radical plastic surgical manoeuvre.

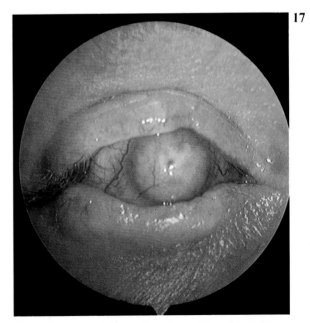

17 Shows outright perforation of the globe following surgical treatment.

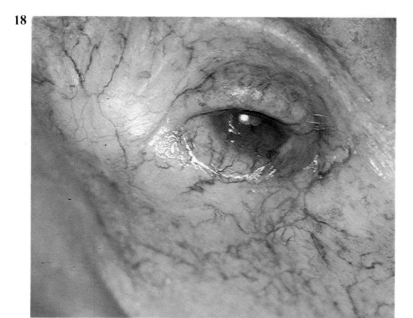

18 Shows severe radiation complications after extensive X-ray therapy.

None of these clinical pictures (Figures 16–18) should be seen nowadays. Radiotherapy seems to be the most satisfactory method, using 'soft' X-rays with full eye protection. (See Figure 27.)

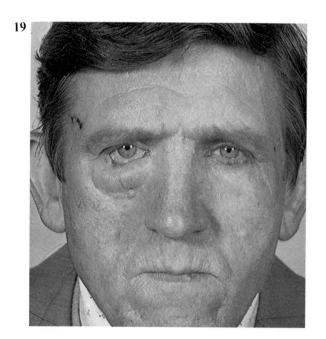

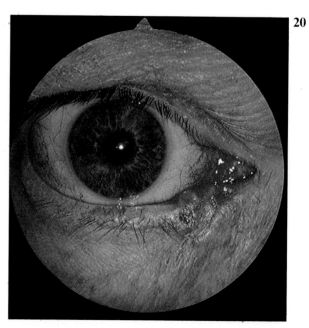

19 (Same case as Figure 16) Shows the unnecessary reconstruction of the right lower eyelid for a proven basal cell carcinoma and the minor side-effects of irradiation, following therapy to a similar lesion on the left lower eyelid.

20 Shows a proven basal cell carcinoma involving the right lower canthus.

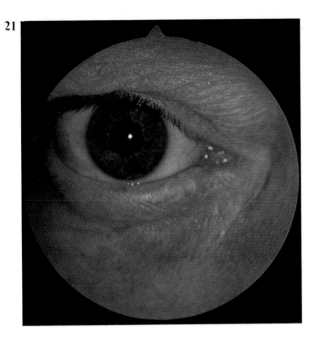

21 Shows the end result of radiotherapy showing depilation of the skin. Other side-effects can be seen but these are of little significance.

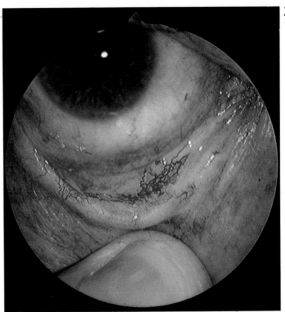

22 Shows conjunctival telangiectasia following a full-thickness dose of irradiation for a proven basal cell carcinoma; this is of no significance. Note that the eye is not involved.

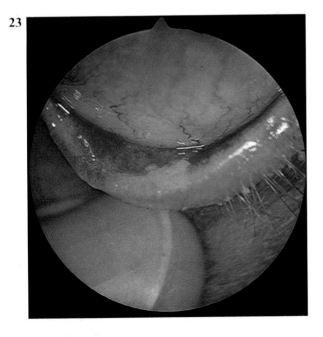

23 Shows a typical 'keratin plaque' on the deep surface of the lid where the irradiation has caused keratinisation of the conjunctival epithelium.

Other skin tumours of a malignant nature, *e.g.* squamous cell carcinomata and, rarely, malignant melanomata are best treated by the same criteria, *i.e.* ascertain the correct diagnosis and then treat with radiotherapy. Ideally, basal cell carcinomata should be followed for five years, squamous cell carcinomata for ten years and other neoplasms indefinitely before a cure can be certain.

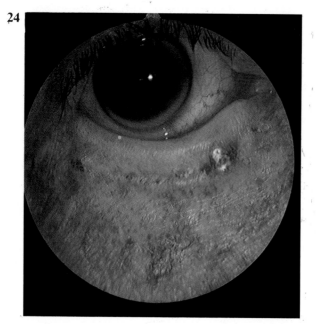

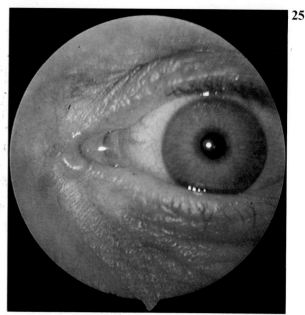

24 Two nodules appearing at either end of a previously irradiated carcinoma. The slightest suspicion of nodularity at any site of a previously treated neoplasm should lead to another biopsy with treatment using non-radiation techniques, *e.g.* excision or cryosurgery (Figures 25 and 26).

25 Shows a small nodule at the inner canthus at an area treated with very high doses of irradiation leading to fibrosis of the lacrimal sac (a complication rarely seen nowadays). This was treated with the insertion of a Lester Jones tube, thus further surgery or radiotherapy was contraindicated.

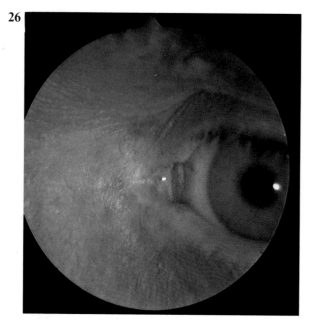

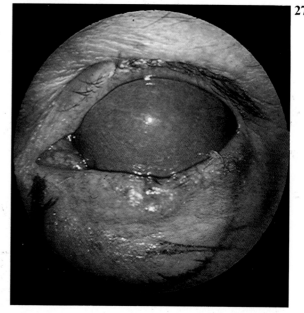

26 Cryosurgery produced a cure.

27 Shows a proven basal cell carcinoma being treated with 'soft' X-rays with full eye protection by a lead shield inserted in the conjunctival sac.

In summary, all skin tumours will need a careful biopsy or a scraping before any precise diagnosis can be established and most cases are probably best treated by 'soft' X-rays with full eye protection (Figure 27), the complications following this being minimal.

Conjunctival tumours

The most emotive, important group is undoubtedly the pigmented lesions, and their diagnosis and management will be discussed in some detail as the criteria for these can be applied easily to other neoplastic or pseudo-neoplastic conditions of the conjunctiva.

PIGMENTED TUMOURS OF THE CONJUNCTIVA

These may be divided into (a) Local and (b) Diffuse.

(a) Local

These neoplasms cannot be differentiated easily from malignant or benign in nature, with a single examination in all cases. In most cases, a period of observation is justified as the benign lesion may become malignant, perhaps over a period of many years. Unless the presence of a black or brown spot concerns the patient (Figure 28) from the cosmetic point of view, no action need be taken unless signs of outright aggression occur. The most common type of benign pigmented lesion (naevus) shows the following features.

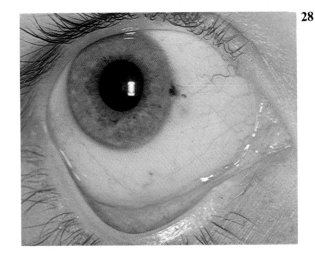

28

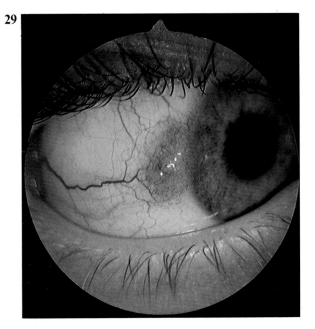

29 It is pigmented, flat or slightly raised with small cysts present below the conjunctiva.

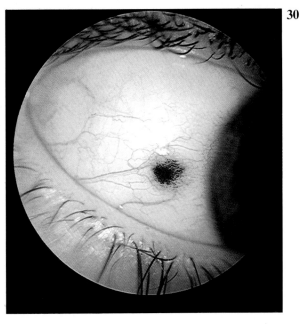

30 Typically they occur at the limbus but may occur elsewhere.

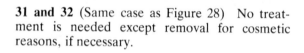

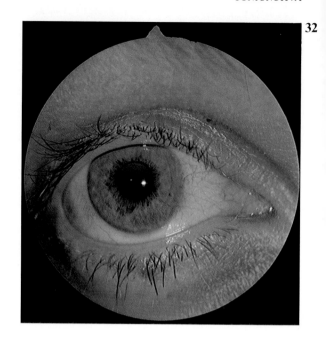

31 and 32 (Same case as Figure 28) No treatment is needed except removal for cosmetic reasons, if necessary.

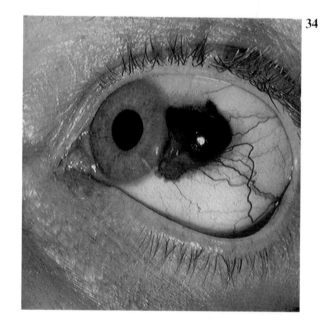

33 and 34 (Same case with a lapse of four years) However, continued observation is necessary as some or, perhaps, all localised malignant melanomata arise from a pre-existing naevus.

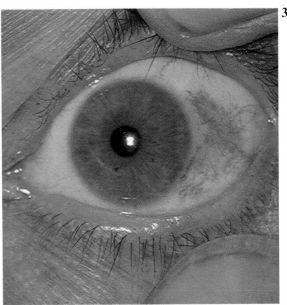

35 A different type of local lesion is that of a 'pre-cancerous' melanosis. These, characteristically, are localised and flat with irregular scattered brownish pigmentation in one area. They may occur at the limbus like a naevus but, also, anywhere else in the conjunctiva, cornea and may involve the skin, merging imperceptibly into the diffuse form of pre-cancerous melanosis.

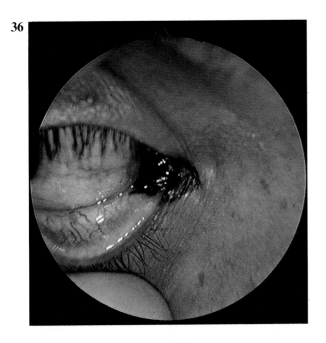

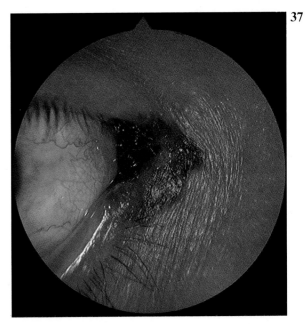

36 and 37 Like a naevus it may undergo malignant change, shown by a period of observation. The fact that a pigmented lesion is malignant may be assumed either from the change from its known previous state, *i.e.* enlargement in area, thickening, the appearance of large feeder vessels, or inflammatory signs.

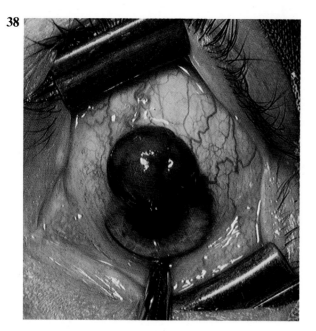

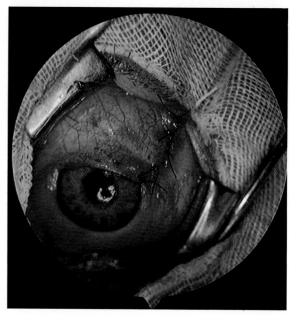

38 The presence of these signs on first examination, however, may also indicate outright malignant change.

39 (Same case as Figures 33 and 34) In either case a careful excisional biopsy of the complete lesion is justified, with the preservation of normal vision.

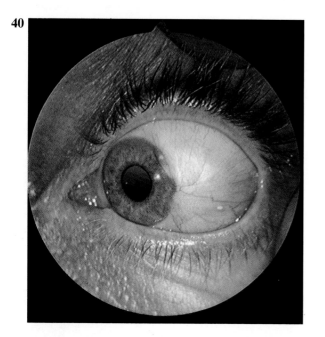

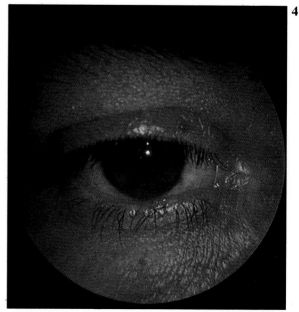

40 (Same case as Figure 39) and **41** (Same case as Figures 36 and 37) Shows excision of localised malignant melanoma with subsequent preservation of eye with normal vision.

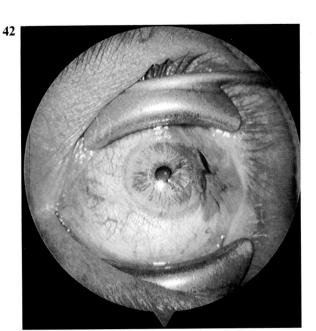

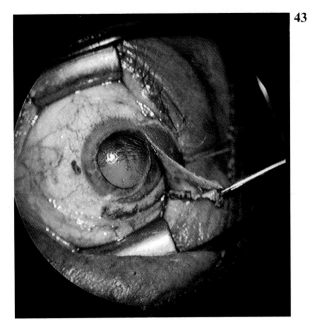

42, 43 and 44 It should be stressed that excision of these lesions must be done very carefully indeed, the plane of dissection going approximately halfway through the cornea and sclera to remove the neoplasm in one piece.

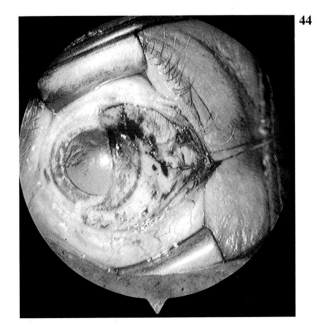

45

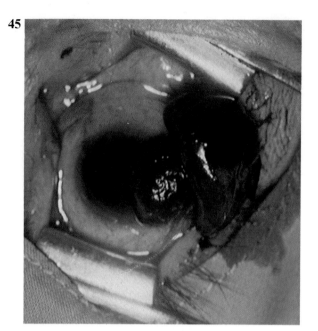

46

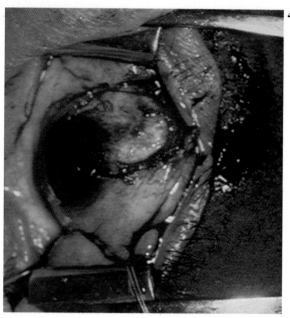

45 Occasionally there may be not only one but, perhaps, two discrete lesions which may become surprisingly raised as they typically rarely penetrate into the globe.

46 (Same case as Figure 45) These types of lesions may be removed successfully locally as they usually have a very narrow pedicle.

47

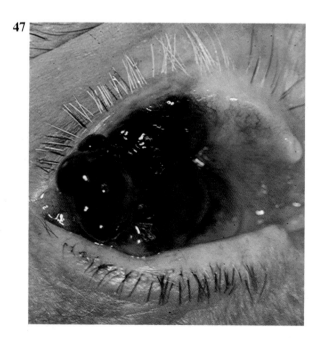

47 Rarely, these lesions occur on a lid where excision of the full-thickness of that part of the lid may be necessary.

(b) Diffuse

Similarly to local pigmented tumours, diffuse tumours cannot be differentiated on a single examination from benign or malignant and, again, in most cases a period of observation is justified.

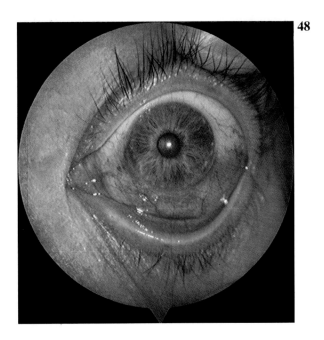

48 The benign lesions are always brownish, speckled, flat, with no inflammatory signs and no large feeder vessels.

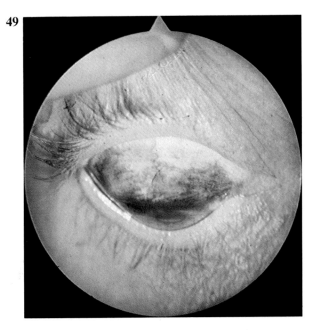

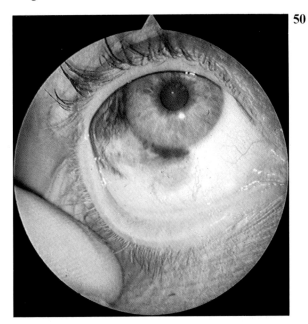

49 and 50 They may involve, however, wide areas of the conjunctiva, cornea and perhaps, even the skin. They may wax and wane, growing larger or smaller as time passes with no malignant propensity.

51

52

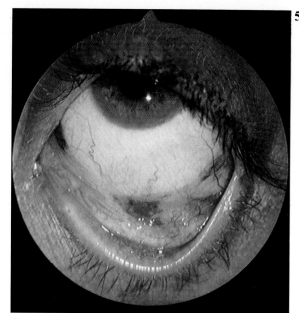

51 and 52 (Same case as Figures 48, 49 and 50) Biopsy should not be undertaken as it may be very difficult for the pathologist to give an accurate opinion and treatment may be unnecessarily precipitated.

53

54

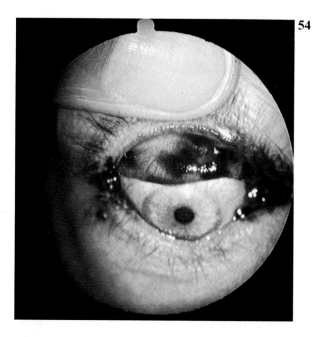

53 and 54 Occasionally, they may become raised or thickened, particularly with pregnancy or after the menopause and after long periods of observation. This change is always characterised by the appearance of thickness, relatively large feeder vessels or inflammatory signs. This patient was observed for sixteen years before such changes appeared. The diffuse changes were biopsied before treatment was undertaken.

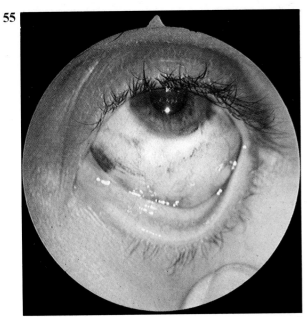

55 The patient had become pregnant on several occasions. On the first occasion the lesion enlarged.

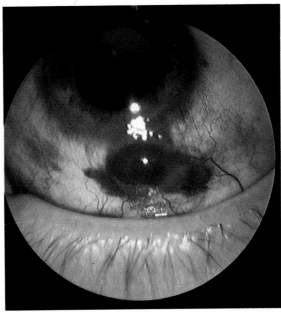

56 On the second occasion a further enlarged area, proven by biopsy to be malignant, was excised with apparent cure. Thus, it would appear that a generalised pre-cancerous melanosis may turn malignant in one small area and, in these cases, localised excisional biopsy may be curative.

57 (Same case as Figures 53 and 54) With these cases, the lids may be split so that the skin may be conserved and the resulting cosmetic appearance is superior to that of classical types of exenteration.

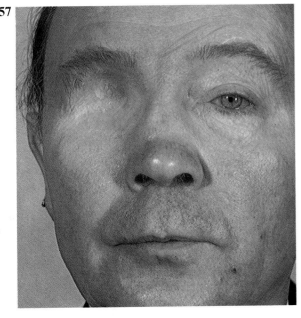

Thus, treatment of the diffuse malignant type can be difficult. If the lesion is flat and on the bulbar conjunctiva or cornea, beta irradiation by a strontium applicator may be effective. If raised, in the fornix or on the back of the lids, exenteration is indicated.

To summarise, most cases of black lesions of the conjunctiva or the skin may be observed. Excisional biopsy of a local lesion may be curative or biopsy of a diffuse lesion is necessary when the lesion has developed large feeder vessels, becomes raised or shows inflammatory signs. In diffuse cases beta irradiation or exenteration may then be needed.

OTHER NEOPLASTIC OR PSEUDO-NEOPLASTIC CONDITIONS OF THE CONJUNCTIVA

(a) Local

58

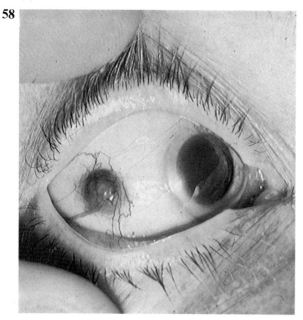

59

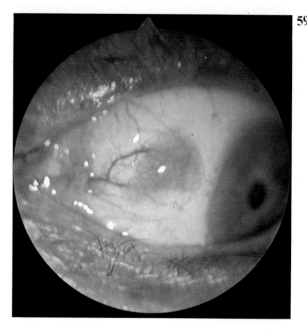

58 Shows a raised brown lump with large feeder vessels. Excision showed the presence of a metallic sub-conjunctival foreign-body.

59 Shows a slowly enlarging, lightly pigmented lesion with large vessels. Histology showed an innocent papilloma.

60

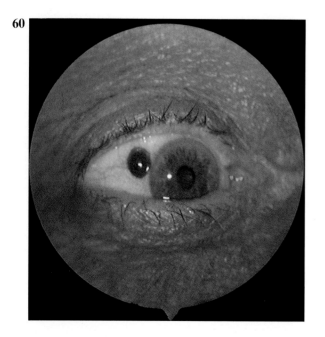

61

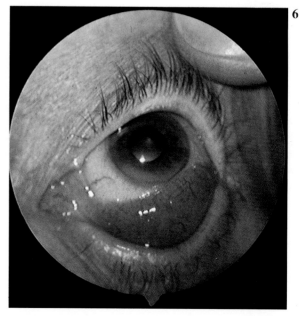

60 The patient complained of a superficial black swelling which was growing larger. Further examination showed a large ciliary body malignant melanoma (with extra-scleral extension).

61 The typical 'salmon-pink' sub-conjunctival swelling characteristic of a lymphoma. They may become bilateral and occasionally are associated with systemic signs of one of the reticulo-sarcomata.

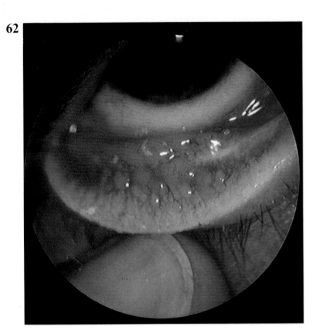

62 The lymphomatous deposits may be aggregated occasionally into small nodules.

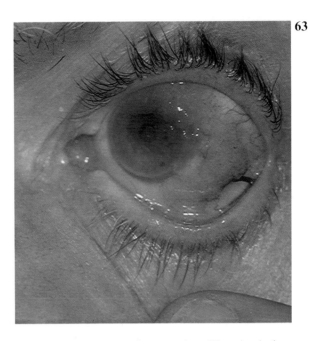

63 Shows a lightly pigmented proliferative lesion. Complete local removal for histology showed a squamous cell carcinoma.

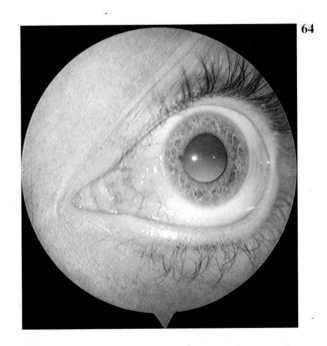

64 Shows a gradually enlarging gelatinous, subconjunctival deposit. Histology showed a leukaematous infiltrate.

(b) Diffuse

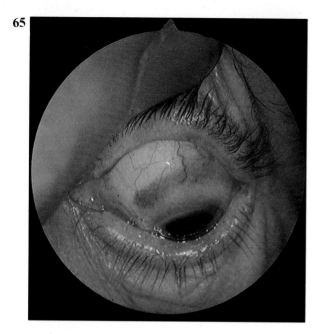

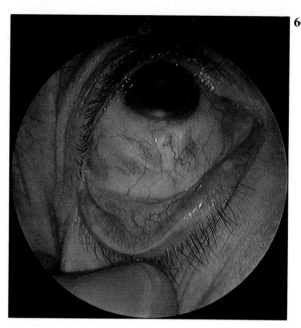

65 and 66 Increased pigment of conjunctiva and iris. Diagnosis – oculodermal melanocytosis. The increased pigment may involve the choroid, the skin of the same side, together with the optic nerve, the bones and even the meninges.

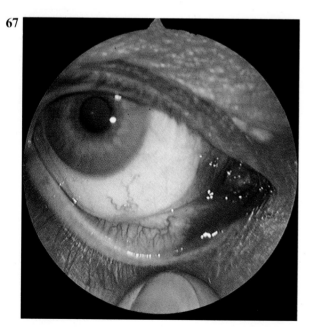

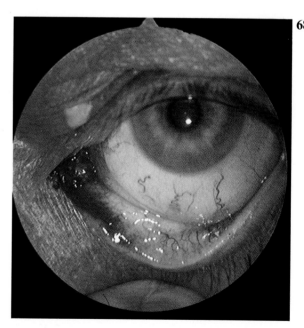

67 and 68 Patient referred with *bilateral* pre-cancerous melanosis. Slit-lamp examination showed silver deposits in the cornea. Occupation – photographic worker. Diagnosis – argyrosis.

69 Showing several rapidly enlarging, pigmented, conjunctival spots with similar ones appearing on the lid margin. Similar spots were seen elsewhere in the skin and the patient died soon afterwards. Diagnosis – secondary malignant melanomata from a primary in the skin of the thigh.

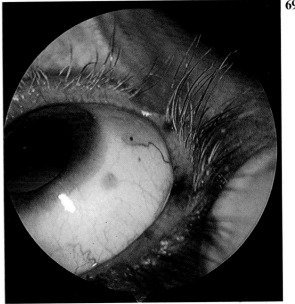

Uveal tumours

Iris tumours

Iris neoplasms again may be sub-divided into malignant and benign. However, it is now known that even the so-called 'malignant' group has an excellent prognosis for life and for many years may be only slowly invasive. In all cases of swellings of the iris where doubt exists as to the diagnosis, a period of observation is justified.

MALIGNANT

A malignant melanoma is the most common tumour seen in this group although the iris is the rarest portion of the uvea to be involved in malignant processes.

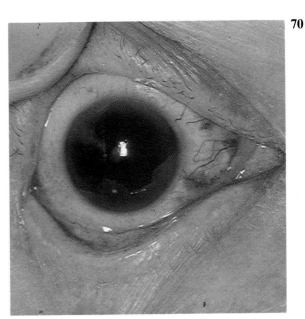

70 The tumour may be flat, diffuse and multi-centric.

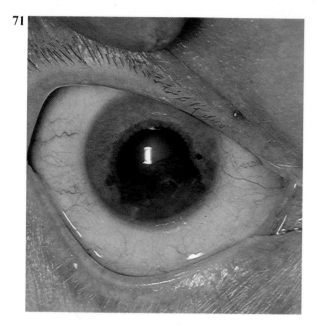

71 The tumour may be solitary and raised.

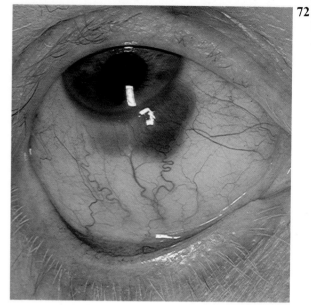

72 They have a propensity to spread around the angle and produce secondary glaucoma; rarely, long-standing lesions may perforate the globe.

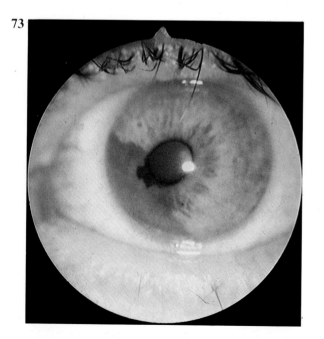

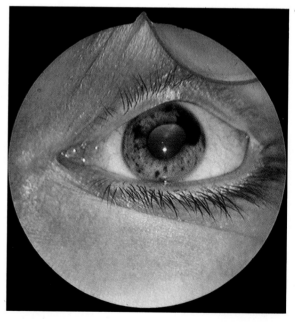

73 and 74 Invariably these lesions are pigmented but sometimes the more rapidly growing tumours appear paler, with a convoluted vascular system. Pupillary distortion is a sign of increasing thickness and usually denotes malignancy.

Such lesions when small are diagnosed easily on a blue iris but may be seen less easily on a brown iris. Wherever there is doubt, observation is all that is needed.

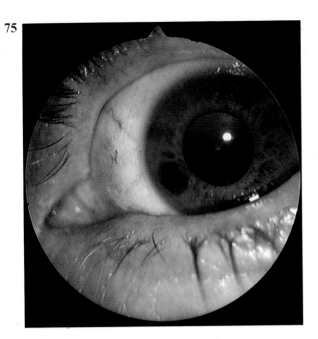

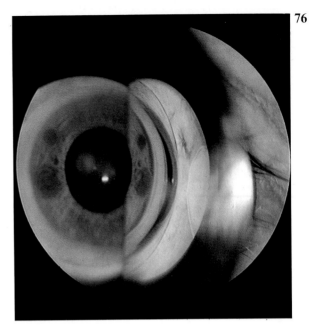

75, 76 and 77 An iridectomy should be done before the tumour involves either the angle or touches the back of the cornea.

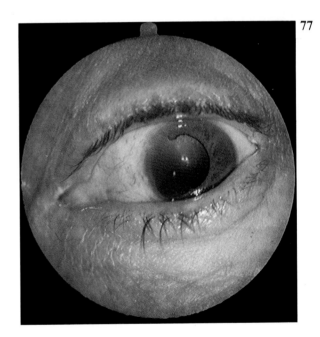

BENIGN

The most common tumour seen is the naevus. It may be flat or, perhaps, slightly thickened, with no vascular system apparent and may be round, linear, single or multiple.

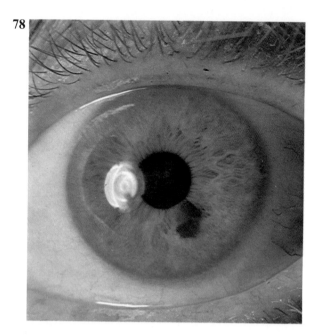

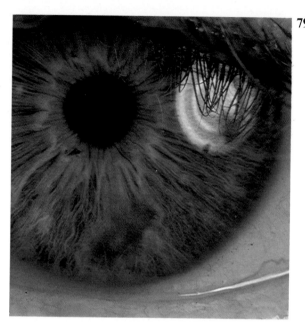

78 The naevus may have well-defined margins, as in this case.

79 In this case the margins are irregular.

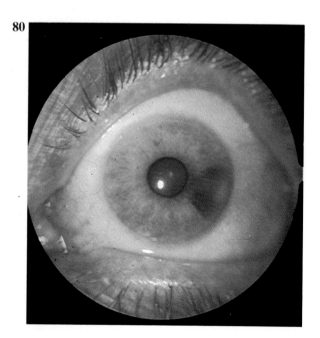

80 A thick iris naevus showing pupillary distortion.

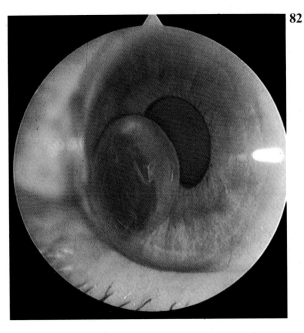

81 Iris cysts are rarer but do not give much difficulty in diagnosis as they are manifestly cystic in appearance.

82 They may be removed easily by puncture and iridectomy if the lesion grows too large.

SECONDARY

These are uncommon and are classically seen from carcinoma of the breast or bronchus but, occasionally, may be noted with other primaries elsewhere.

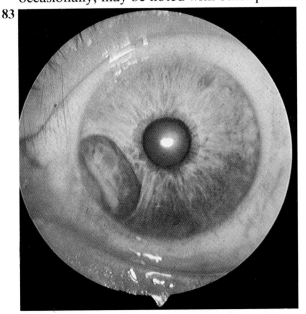

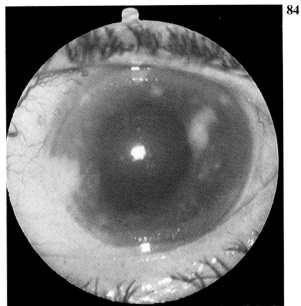

83 Shows a single metastasis but they may be multiple. They are rapidly growing and may show little cell cohesion so the malignant cells appear to be freely circulating in the aqueous.

84 There is consequent blockage of the angle, producing secondary glaucoma and external irradiation is indicated.

Ciliary body tumours

The most common ciliary body tumours of clinical significance are of a malignant nature, while the benign neoplasms are small and rarely enlarge to give symptoms. Unfortunately, this is also true of malignant tumours at the beginning of their growth. They never give symptoms until they grow outside the confines of the ciliary body.

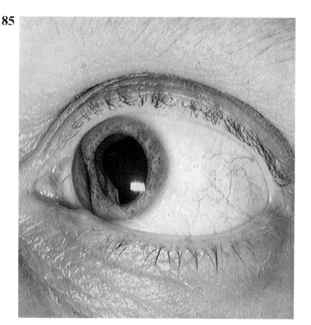

85 Showing a relatively small ciliary body neoplasm passing *forwards* with large anterior extension.

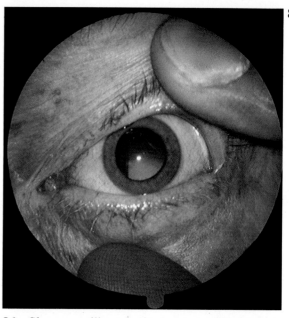

86 Shows a ciliary body tumour with *inwards* extension pressing and distorting the lens.

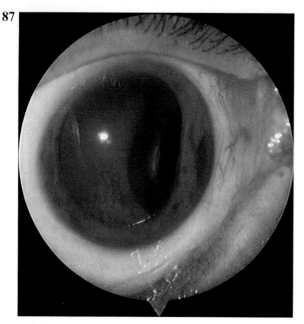

87 Further progression may give rise to lens opacities.

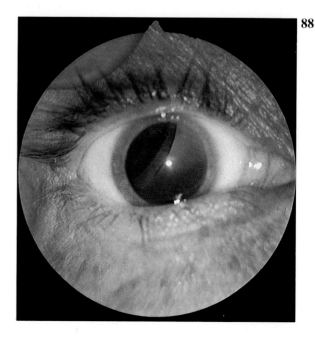

88 Shows the tumour passing *backwards* under the ora when a serous detachment may then occur posteriorly, producing visual changes.

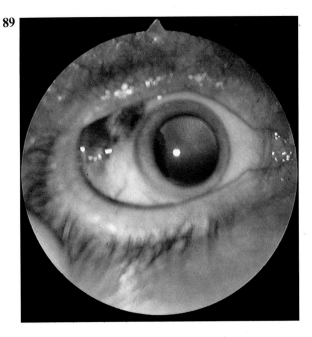

89 Shows a large ciliary body tumour which had spread *outwards* so that the patient complained of a visible dark swelling on the outside of the eye.

All these stages represent a ciliary body tumour which is beyond the state of cyclectomy and conservative surgical cure and enucleation is indicated.

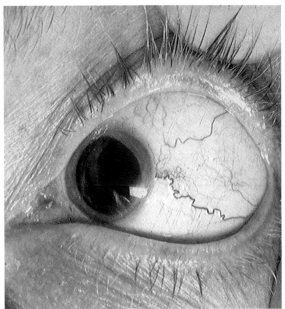

90 Small ciliary body tumours which may be removed locally should be suspected by a triad of signs: loss of vision, slight hypotony and a 'sentinel vein'.

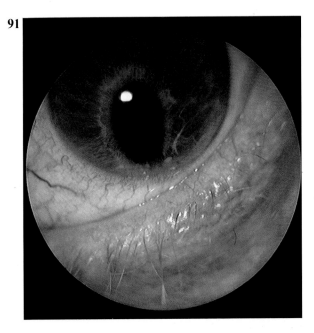

91 Other progressive lesions of the ciliary body are rare but should be borne in mind, *e.g.* a secondary tumour which has produced retraction of the iris, the primary being in the breast.

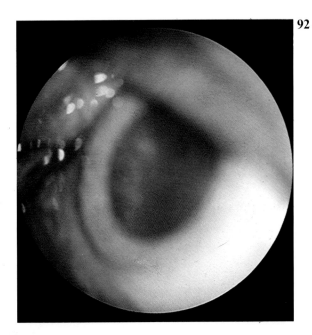

92 Shows a ciliary body melanocytoma with extra-scleral extension. The extension outwards was biopsied and the diagnosis confirmed. (Child aged five.) (See Figure 113.)

Choroid

INTRODUCTION

Choroidal malignant melanomata are the most common, albeit still rather rare, intra-ocular tumours that are met in clinical practice. There is now no doubt that they grow relatively slowly and any doubt as to diagnosis justifies a period of observation. These tumours will be considered under three headings:

1 Physical signs

    (a) Typical malignant melanomata arbitrarily divided into:
        (i) early
        (ii) medium
        (iii) late
    (b) Rarer types of presentations

2 Differential diagnoses

    (a) Flat lesions
    (b) Lesions with a serous retinal detachment
    (c) Rarer lesions

3 Appearances after conservative therapy

    (a) Successful treatment
    (b) Complications

1 PHYSICAL SIGNS

(a) Typical malignant melanomata

(i) Early

These early tumours are either symptomless and, therefore, noticed at a routine eye examination, or else appear at or near the macula producing distortion of vision.

93

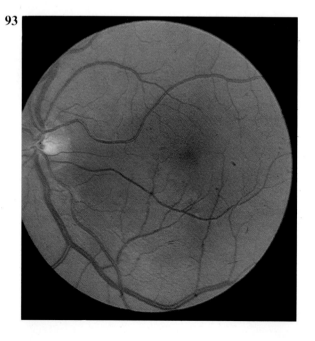

93 Shows a very early flat grey lesion with ill-defined edges, but one or two orange-coloured patches are seen on the nasal margin. Naevi are often darker, with well-defined feathered edges with small white circular areas on their surfaces (colloid bodies – see Figure 111). These 'orange patches', and not the paler ones seen on naevi, are characteristic of malignant melanomata and in this case a fluorescein angiogram confirmed the diagnosis. Such flat tumours are easily treated by light-coagulation (see Figure 120).

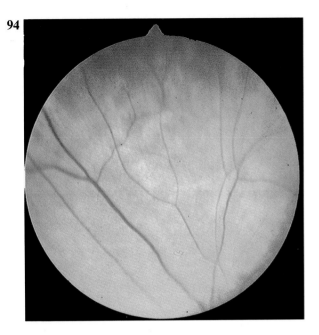

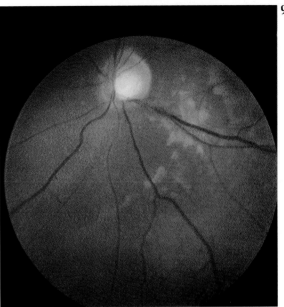

94 Shows a larger malignant melanoma with typical 'orange patches' which are pathognomonic of this type of malignant melanoma. Although flat, a tumour of this size probably cannot be treated conservatively. These 'orange patches' are deposits of lipofuschin in the pigment epithelium, and therefore are never seen on the raised 'collar-stud' portion of a larger malignant melanoma which has perforated Bruch's membrane.

95 A large, flat posterior malignant melanoma. Note the 'orange patches' which developed, during a period of observation, on a pre-existing naevus. This malignant change is well known and, ideally, all naevi should be assessed regularly and appropriate treatment instigated if malignant characteristics develop (indeed, it may be that all malignant melanomata develop from a pre-existing innocent naevus).

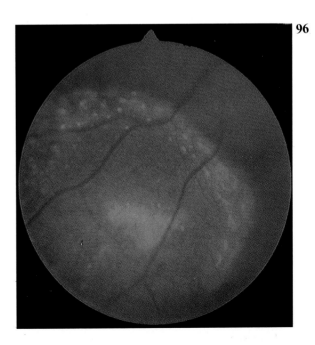

96 This tumour is becoming raised and rounded but, as yet, has not extended through Bruch's membrane. Note the classical 'orange patches'. There is, however, a slight overlying serous detachment suggesting that perforation of Bruch's membrane and the pigment epithelium is imminent.

(ii) Medium

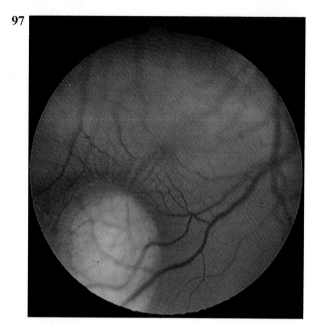

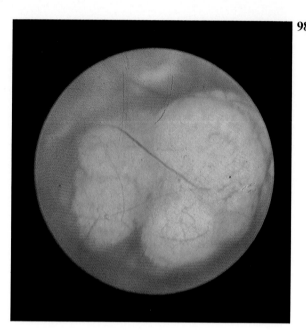

97 Shows a malignant melanoma with an extension through Bruch's membrane and the pigment epithelium characterised by a white, raised area (the top of the 'collar-stud') with a secondary circulation in it. Typically the extension, as in this case, is not pigmented and the darker flat basement portion of the earlier type of tumour can be seen around the edge of the lower plane.

98 The 'collar-stud' may grow larger and larger, still staying typically non-pigmented with vessels coursing through its substance. As it grows larger the base of the original tumour may not be seen easily. Eyes containing this type of neoplasm are best enucleated.

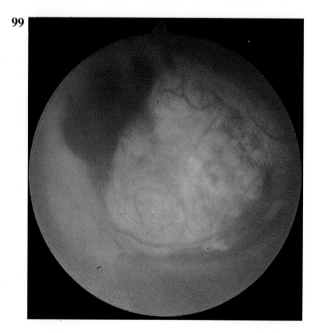

99 Occasionally, such extensions produce haemorrhage on its surface or around the base.

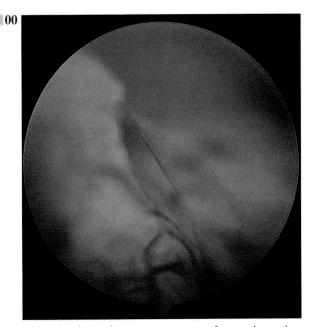

100 At times the tumour may perforate the retina into the vitreous. In this photograph the edge of the retina may be seen passing obliquely across the waist of the neoplasm. Obviously, enucleation is the only feasible form of therapy.

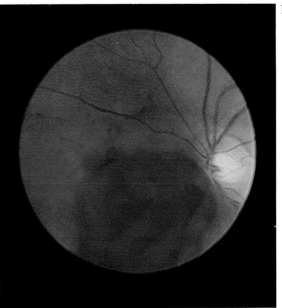

101 Less commonly, such extensions inwards through Bruch's membrane and the pigment epithelium are densely pigmented but still exhibit the same characteristics of relatively slow growth in all planes.

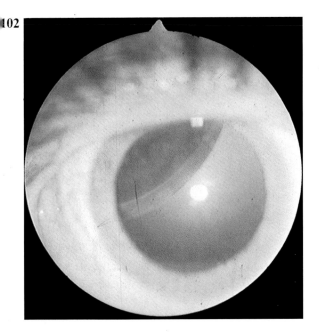

102 Rarely, the tumour does not produce a 'collar-stud' type of architecture but remains sessile, growing larger and larger over a long period of time. In this case a peripheral choroidal melanoma has passed under the ora serrata to involve the ciliary body.

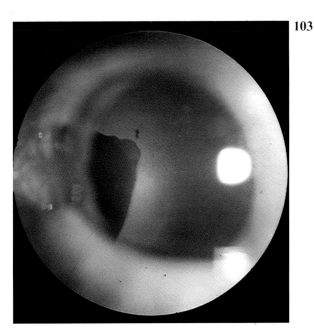

103 Sometimes these larger sessile tumours may break off small groups of tumour cells into the vitreous.

(iii) Late

104

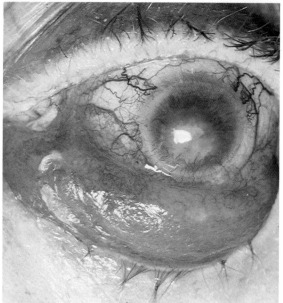

105

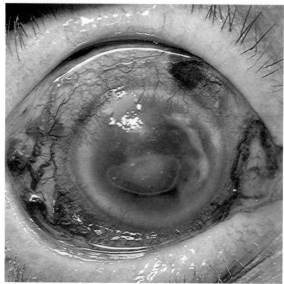

104   The end result of a long-standing choroidal malignant melanoma which has filled the eye, producing glaucoma, and perforated the globe, producing proptosis.

105   Shows the end result of an eye which has received several glaucoma operations in an attempt to reduce the pressure in a blind eye with a rubeosis of the iris: the diagnosis being presumed to be that of a central retinal vein thrombosis. The dark areas seen are not staphylomata but are extra-scleral extensions of the tumour.

Any eye which has an insidious loss of vision with a rubeosis of the iris and secondary glaucoma should be presumed to harbour a tumour unless proved otherwise (*e.g.* by ultrasonics if the media is opaque).

(b) Rarer types of presentations

106

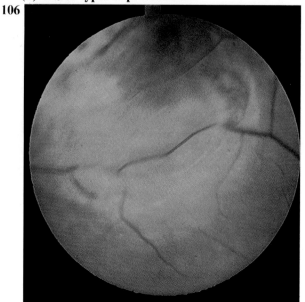

107

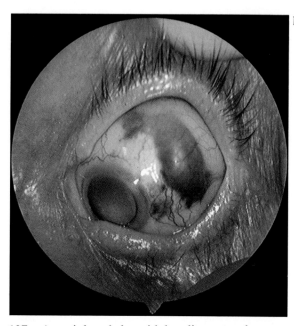

106   Showing a 'U'-shaped tear on the summit of a medium-sized malignant melanoma: note the 'orange patches' below the lower margin of the tear. At one time it was taught that the presence of a retinal break precluded the presence of a tumour.

107   A peripheral choroidal malignant melanoma presenting with extrascleral extension, together with involvement of the ciliary body.

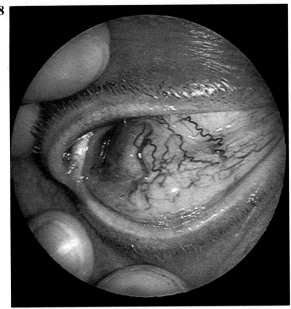

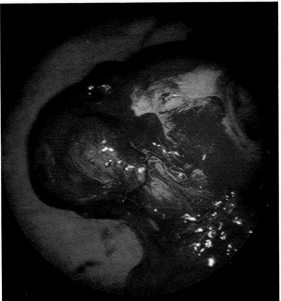

108 A rare type of presentation. A sub-conjunctival lump presented in the lower fornix, the eye appearing apparently normal. Biopsy of the sub-conjunctival mass showed the typical structure of a choroidal malignant melanoma. Further re-examination of the eye showed no intra-ocular abnormality.

109 (Same case as Figure 108)   The anterior half of the orbit was exenterated, when a large malignant melanoma was seen adherent to the sclera, histologically arising from within a scleral canal.

2 DIFFERENTIAL DIAGNOSES

(a) Flat lesions, corresponding approximately with the early group of malignant melanomata featured above

(b) Lesions with an overlying serous retinal detachment   (c) Rarer lesions

(a) Flat lesions

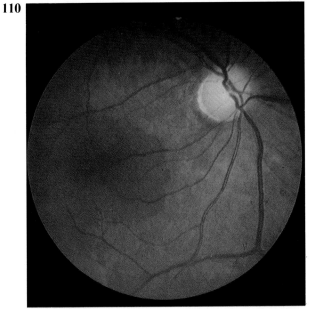

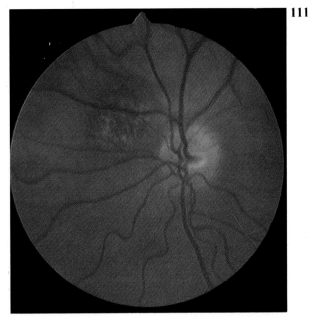

110 Shows a classical naevus which is usually the most common error in diagnosis. It is small, dark, flat with feathered edges and characteristically at the posterior pole. Such cases need infrequent follow-up.

111 Sometimes a naevus shows small rounded, fairly well-defined yellow or white patches which are colloid bodies (not 'orange patches', see above). Such cases need only infrequent observation to exclude a malignant change.

112

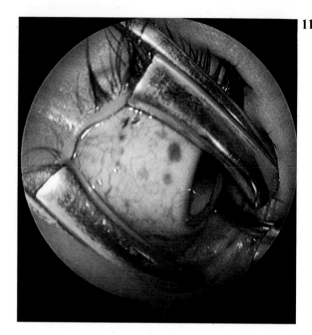

113

112 Shows a small densely pigmented juxta-papillary tumour; the classical site for a melano-cytoma.

113 Rarely, melanocytomata may occur anteriorly as in this case, producing extra-scleral extension (proven by histology), no change being noticed over five years. Thus, the presence of pigmented patches outside the eye, confluent with a dark intra-ocular swelling does not necessarily indicate the presence of a malignant melanoma.

114

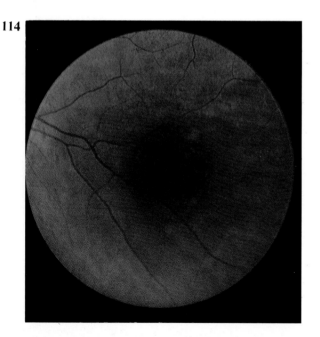

115

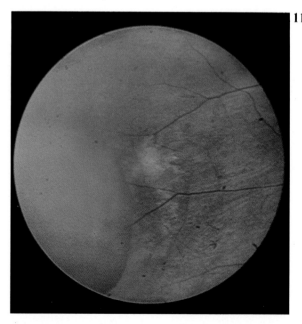

114 and 115 Shows a flat, rounded, densely pigmented lesion with the suspicion of a clear halo on its edge. This is characteristic of congenital hyperplasia of the pigmented epithelium. No treatment is needed.

(b) Serous retinal lesions (corresponding to those tumours with extensions through Bruch's membrane)

Since the advent of the routine use of indirect ophthalmoscopy, it is highly unlikely that a retinal detachment, even with a hole (see Figure 106), will mask an underlying intra-ocular malignant melanoma. This is largely a theoretical hazard in terms of differential diagnosis.

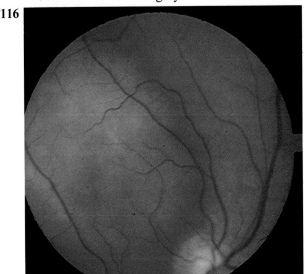

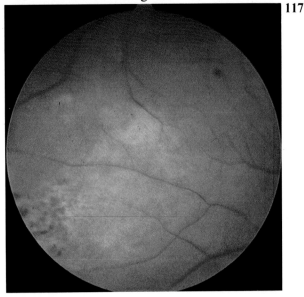

116 Shows a typical choroidal metastasis (from a carcinoma of the breast). These neoplasms are pale with fluffy ill-defined margins, perhaps with an overlying serous retinal detachment. They may be bilateral and/or multiple in one eye.

117 Shows a raised, pinkish sub-retinal mass with densely convoluted vessels, the overlying retina showing a marked cystoid change. This is the classical appearance of an haemangioma, treatment being light-coagulation.

(c) Rarer lesions

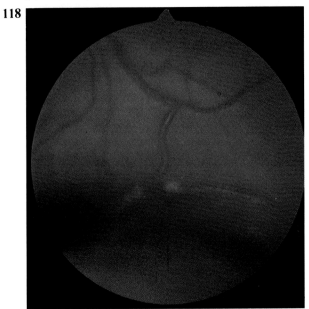

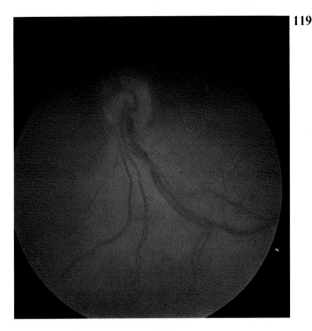

118 and 119 Show a very darkly pigmented sub-retinal mass with large draining retinal veins. Histology showed a carcinoma of the pigment epithelium. This is a very rare condition and should

be suspected when the tumour is densely pigmented and surrounded with large vessels. Rarely, a malignant melanoma of the choroid may simulate this appearance, *i.e.* a 'retinal haemangioma'.

3 APPEARANCES AFTER CONSERVATIVE THERAPY

(a) Successful treatment

The initial work for the conservative treatment of intra-ocular tumours entailed the use of radioactive cobalt discs emitting gamma radiation, and this is still the standard technique used in England. Elsewhere in the world other gamma emitters are used, *e.g.* gold, while other centres use beta emitters, *e.g.* ruthenium. All these techniques can be successful in certain carefully selected cases, so that examples of satisfactory tumour regression will be shown. It is equally certain, however, that the improper use of nearly all these types of beta or gamma emitters will produce the same (sometimes catastrophic) side-effects. It is considered in order to illustrate some of these complications. The present indications for each form of therapy will not be discussed.

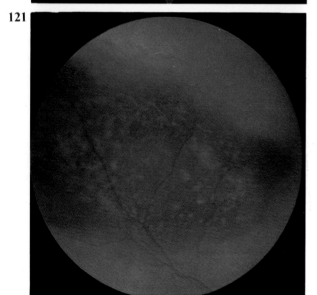

120 There is no doubt that light-coagulation may produce a cure in certain flat early tumours, as in this case. It is of no use applying light to large tumours or those with any appreciable thickness, as it is impossible to eradicate all the tumour cells.

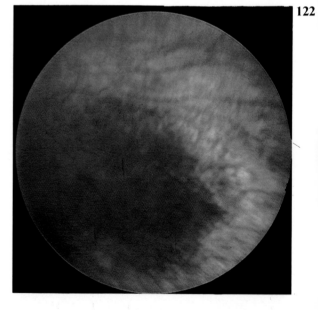

121 Shows an early malignant melanoma, slightly thick with 'orange patches' and no extension through Bruch's membrane. As the tumour was not adjacent to the optic nerve (see later), a cobalt plaque was applied.

122 Shows the same case six months later. There is thinning of the lesion, secondary depigmentation of the retina and atrophy of the choroid occurring around the edge of the tumour.

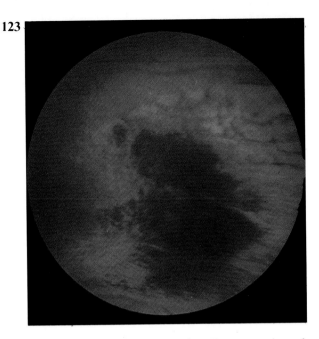

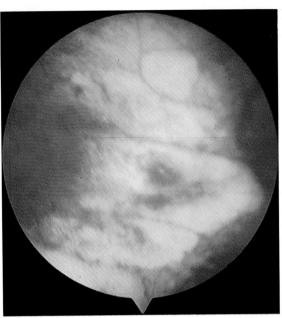

123 (Same case as Figure 121) The regression of the tumour is virtually complete with much choroido-retinal atrophy around its edge. The continuation of this regression may take up to two years to develop, as in this case.

124 (Same case as Figure 121) The choroidal atrophy continues for years (in this case, four years) after the application of a radioactive disc or plaque.

It seems likely that the tumour regression is so slow that it is dependent on *vascular* changes *induced* by the irradiation. It is because of these vascular changes that severe complications may develop when the large retinal vessels are irradiated (see below).

(b) Complications

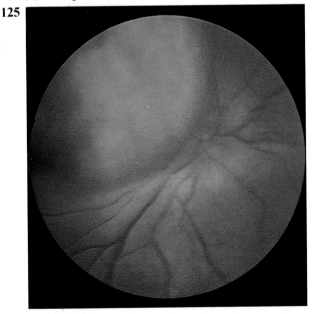

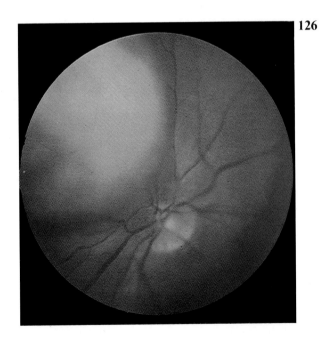

125 Shows a medium-sized, sessile, juxta-papillary malignant melanoma. A cobalt plaque was applied.

126 (Same case as Figure 125) Seven months later, there are signs of tumour regression as evidenced by some shrinkage in the bulk of the neoplasm.

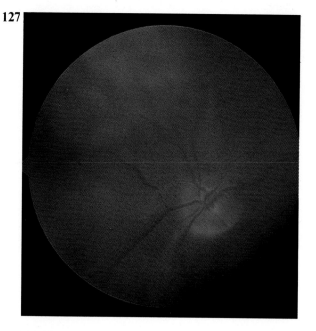

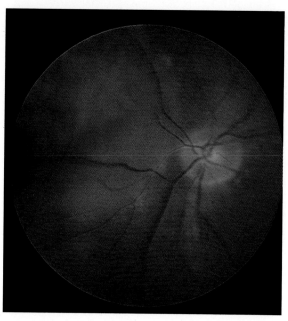

127 (Same case as Figure 125) Nine months after the application of a plaque, there is obvious reduction in the mass of the neoplasm.

128 (Same case as Figure 125) Shows further regression eleven months after the irradiation.

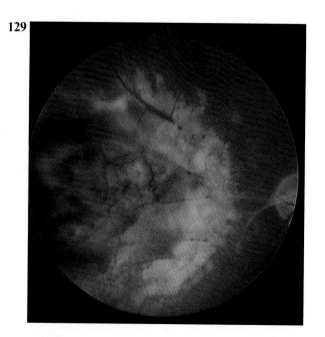

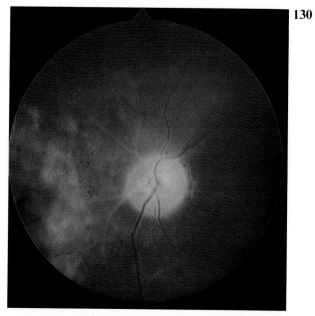

129 (Same case as Figure 125) The tumour continues to regress to a flat scar.

130 (Same case as Figure 125) One year after the application of a plaque. The patient awoke with no perception of light in this eye due to an acute vascular insufficiency of the optic nerve, presumably radiation-induced.

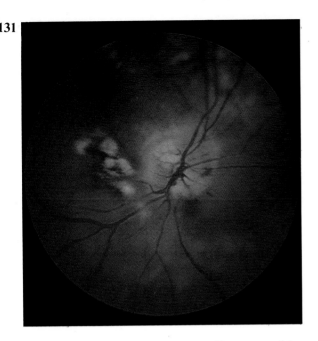

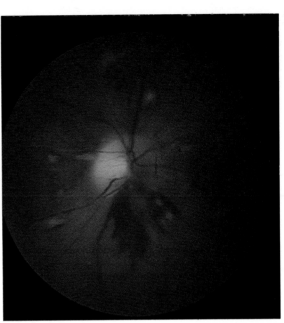

131 Shows other severe side-effects: notably, occlusion of blood vessels, juxta-papillary haemorrhages and exudates with severe loss of vision consequent on a radiation source applied adjacent to the optic nerve.

132 Juxta-papillary haemorrhages and exudates may occur even when the source of radiation may be some distance away from the optic nerve, as in this case.

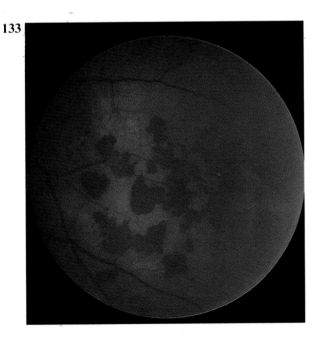

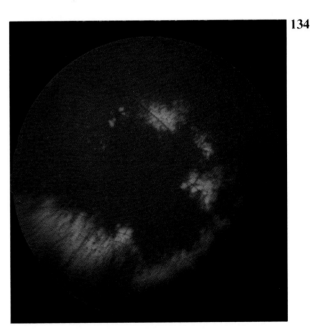

133 Occasionally the haemorrhages may occur in the retina in a quadrant opposite to the area treated, as in this case.

134 In addition to the haemorrhage, there may occur a 'circinate' type of retinopathy even in young patients, when focal irradiation is attempted near the optic nerve or macula.

135

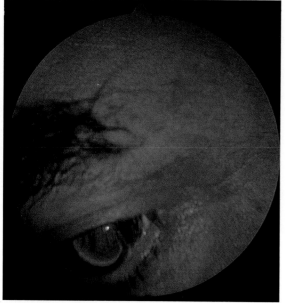

135 Some complications may be seen externally as in this case, where there was a permanent loss of the hair of the eyebrow close to a plaque placed supra-temporally, the radiation coming from the back of the plaque.

136

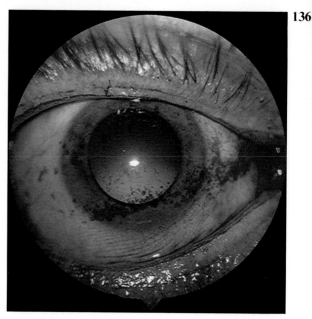

136 In this case the application of a plaque supra-temporally induced a 'dry eye' because of the radiation from the back of the plaque affecting the lacrimal gland.

137

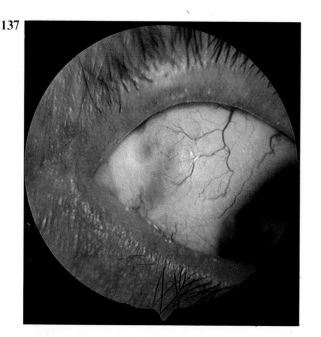

137 It is highly likely that all cases treated with a radioactive disc or plaque, from whatever source, develop scleral necrosis which will only manifest itself when the tumour is anterior, as in this case.

138

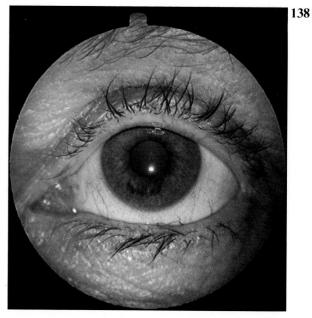

138 A large plaque was placed against the sclera to irradiate a tumour inferiorly. Years later, iris atrophy became apparent.

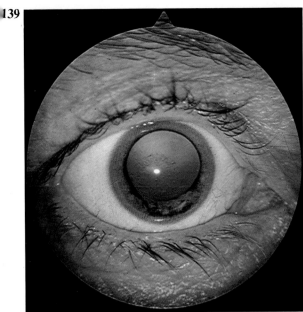

139 (Same case as Figure 138) Shows progression of the iris atrophy and the very earliest signs of a radiation cataract.

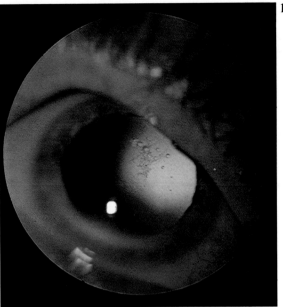

140 Occasionally, even a radioactive plaque or disc placed posteriorly may induce a radiation-induced cataract anteriorly of a minor nature, as in this case, merely being a few non-progressive globules in the posterior portion of the lens.

141 There is no place for the deliberate irradiation of a whole eye with *external* irradiation techniques, as opposed to focal methods previously described. The dose of gamma rays necessary to achieve a tumourcidal level will lead to xerophthalmia, cataract and glaucoma. This eye was treated by this method for a large tumour and was subsequently enucleated because of pain. The tumour was found to be inert histologically but, clearly, it is not a feasible form of therapy.

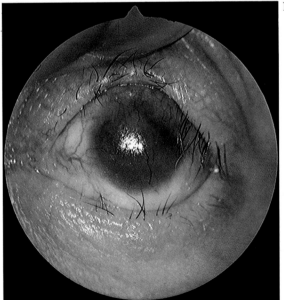

Retinal tumours – retinoblastoma

INTRODUCTION

Retinoblastoma are excessively rare, so that many clinicians may only see one or two cases in a lifetime. It is because of this that sometimes the clinical diagnosis is delayed, or doubt exists as to the efficacy of any therapy linked with an incomplete knowledge of the side-effects of therapy. To this end, the tumour will be shown in its varying degrees of severity ranging from the symptom-free to certain death, together with the various types of regression and side-effects after treatment.

1 PHYSICAL SIGNS

(a) Early

The earliest forms of retinoblastoma may be seen when a child is 'at risk', *i.e.* a sibling of an affected child or the progeny of an affected parent, is being examined early after birth with no clinical symptoms apparent.

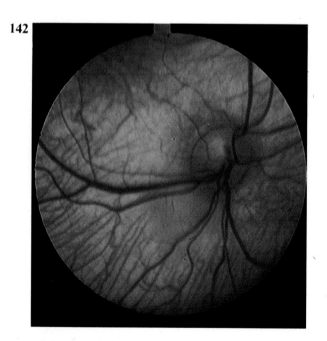

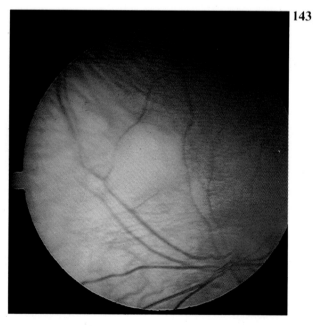

142 A small tumour appears 1 mm in diameter and is apparent below the optic disc, only distinguishing itself by a slight blurring of the choroidal pattern underneath.

143 Shows a slightly larger tumour showing more obvious characteristics of thickness and pinkness due to the presence of many small vessels.

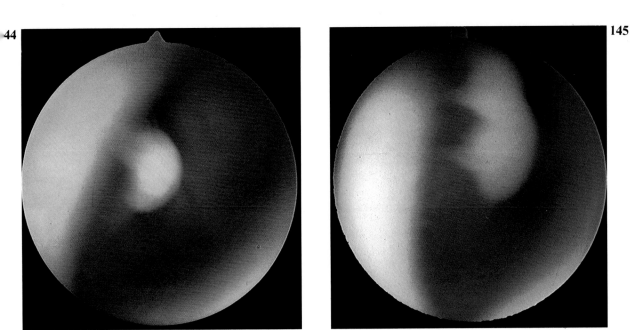

144 Obviously, these small tumours can be very peripheral and may be seen only with the technique of binocular ophthalmoscopy and scleral depression, as in this case.

145 Shows a slightly larger tumour only visible with scleral depression. The tumour is passing forwards across the base of the ora serrata.

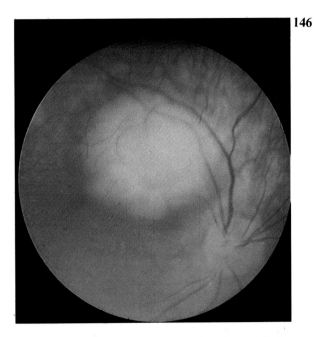

146 A larger tumour with slightly enlarged draining veins, the densely white surface of fine blood vessels being more apparent.

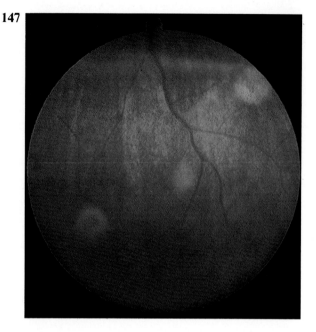

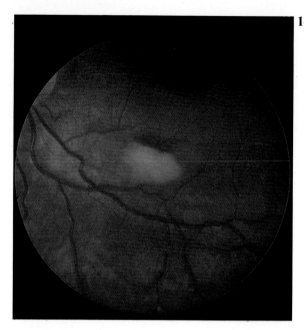

147 Occasionally, new neoplasms may arise from a previously treated primary and grow larger as time passes (three diaphanous 'cannon-ball' tumours suspended in the vitreous).

148 (Same case as Figure 147) The tumours are becoming thicker and larger but still floating within the globe.

These cases are impossible to treat by focal means and, if the whole eye has been treated before, these tumours must be left to proliferate when vision may then drop and the eye can be removed with no danger to the child. It must be emphasised that it may take *months* to demonstrate these changes, so that periods of observation are justifiable.

(b) Medium

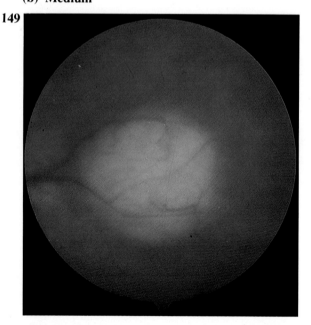

149 Shows a medium-sized neoplasm with fine blood vessels, a whitish body and large draining veins (a constant feature of retinoblastomata).

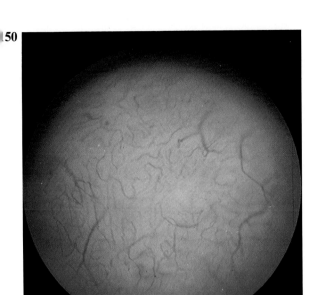

150 The typical surface of a medium-sized retinoblastoma. White, raised with fine blood vessels coursing over its surface. However, a portion of it can break into the vitreous (Figure 152), when the appearances are very different.

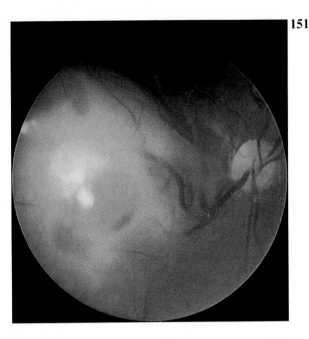

151 Occasionally, cystic changes appear within the substance of a medium-sized neoplasm (note the large draining veins).

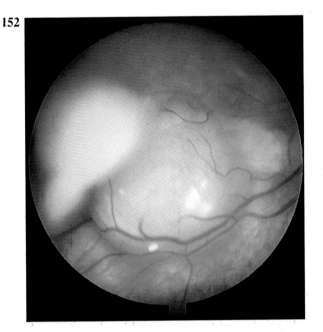

152 Shows a sessile retinal neoplasm with a white, fluffy, vascular portion which has spread into the vitreous as a diffuse floating fluffy white cloud.

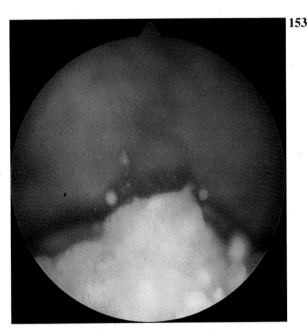

153 Occasionally, the mass of tumour breaking off into the vitreous is not fluffy, but is more aggregated as seen here (Figures 161 and 162 are examples of a later stage of such process).

154

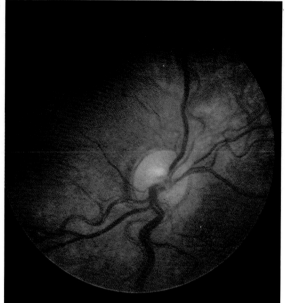

155

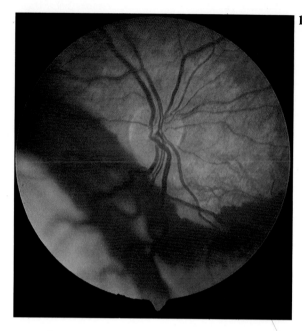

154 (Same case as Figure 153) Note the large draining veins (examples of which have been noted in Figures 149 and 151). At times these large feeder vessels may suggest the diagnosis of a vascular tumour, *e.g.* haemangioma; however, many retinoblastomata show these large draining veins.

155 Early retinal haemorrhage may occur and the edge of the medium tumour may show areas of haemorrhage.

(c) Large

156

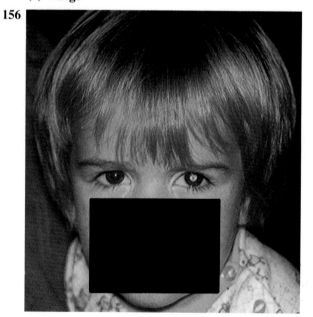

157

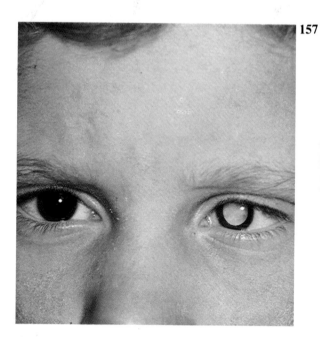

156 Larger tumours, perhaps the first in a generation, may be noted in a family photograph as a classical white pupil.

157 Shows the classical signs of a white pupil and a squint.

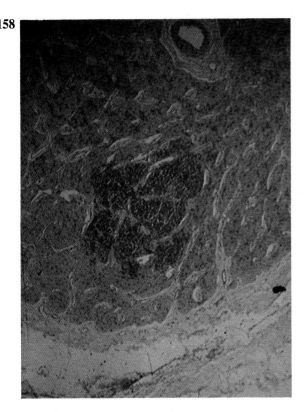

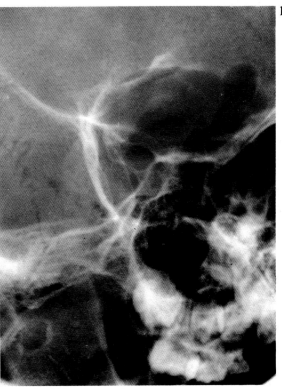

158 (Same case as Figure 157)   The tumour has invaded the optic nerve.

159 (Same case as Figure 157)   The tumour has passed up the optic nerve and has enlarged the optic foramen.

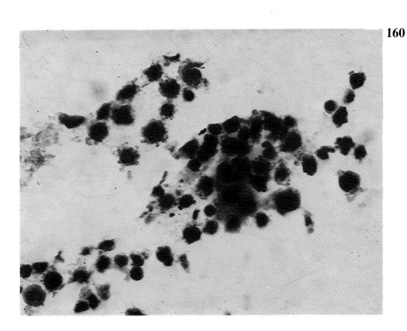

160 (Same case as Figure 157)   The tumour can then spread to the cerebro-spinal fluid. It must be emphasised that tumours of this type are very long-standing and must have been present for a long period of time.

161

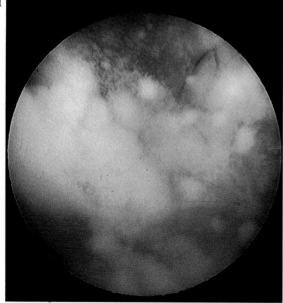

162

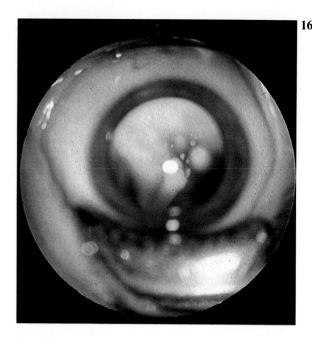

161 (Same case as Figure 147)   Small recurrences may have to be left and grow within the vitreous as confluent (Figure 162) or spherical (Figure 165) tumour masses.

162 (Same case as Figure 161)   In this case, the eye has filled up with a virtually confluent mass of tumour cells.

163

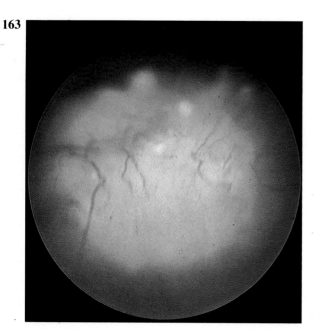

164

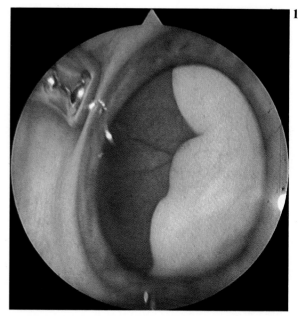

163   At other times, these larger tumours remain localised within the retina, with many fine blood vessels and some calcified plaques being apparent within the main tumour bulk.

164   These retinal tumours may grow larger and remain solid, growing and filling the eye.

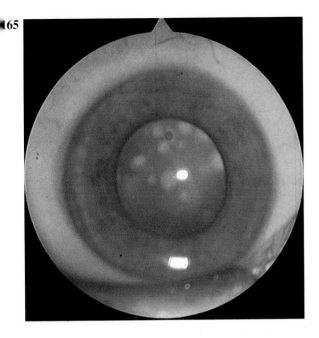

165 Shows floating solid spherical separate masses of tumour floating round within the vitreous.

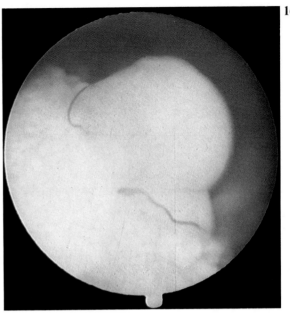

166 At other times these larger tumours are composed of a retinal mass (below and to the left) and a vitreous portion (above and to the right).

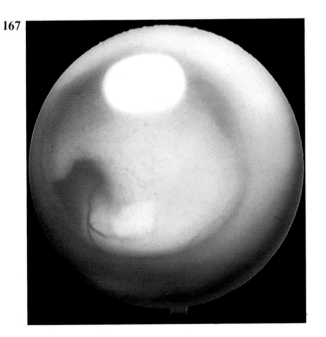

167 A sessile type of larger tumour showing the sessile retinal portion below and to the right with a curved vitreous portion to the left and above.

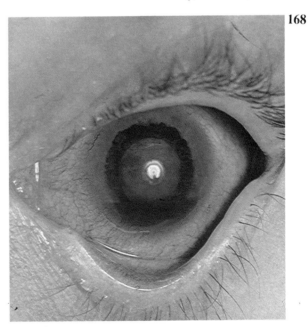

168 Rarely a retinoblastoma presents as a disorganised eye with an hyphaema.

169

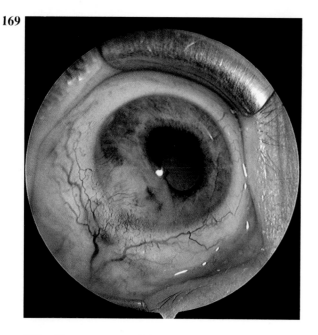

170

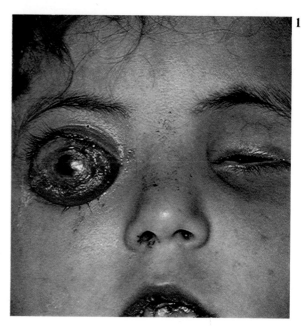

169 Shows a rare iris recurrence of a retinoblastoma in an eye previously treated for a larger sessile retinal type of retinoblastoma.

170 Shows a later stage in an advanced retinoblastoma with proptosis due to extra-ocular extension.

2 DIFFERENTIAL DIAGNOSES

(a) Congenital
(b) Acquired

All the following conditions were referred with a diagnosis of retinoblastoma.

(a) Congenital

171

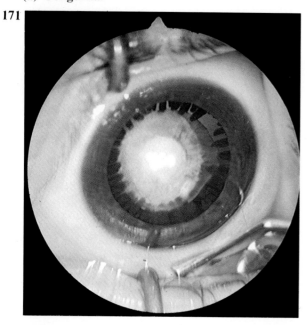

171 Persistent primary hyperplastic vitreous. Typically occurring in a microphthalmic eye, the lens opacity appears white which gives the superficial appearance of a 'cat's eye' reflex. On full examination, the opacity can be seen to occupy a great portion of the lens as in this case or, sometimes, merely a small plaque posteriorly. The long ciliary processes are pathognomonic.

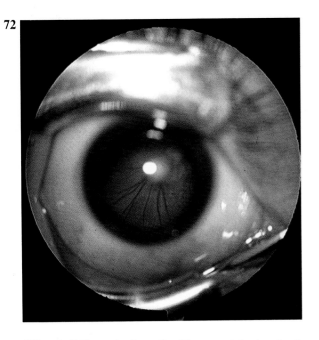

172 A 'Mittendorf spot' with a persistent patent hyaloid system and a traction detachment.

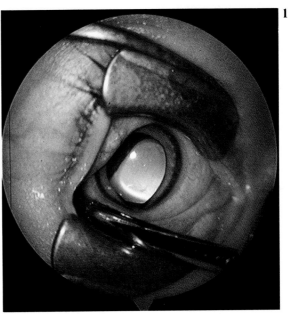

173 A large coloboma of the choroid (and the iris) showing as a white pupil.

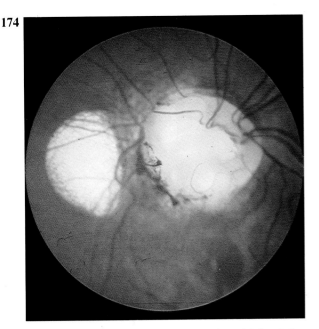

174 A smaller coloboma of the choroid (and the disc) giving the illusion of a sessile retinoblastoma.

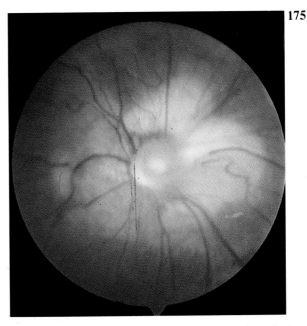

175 A 'Morning Glory' syndrome showing the typical raised pigmented area around the disc with abberant retinal vessels coursing over it. (These occur in one eye and may be associated with an encephalocoele at the base of the skull.) Rarely a coloboma of the choroid may occur in the same eye or the fellow eye.

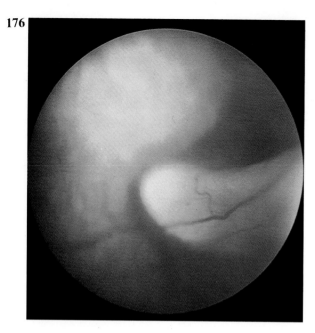

176 Other disc abnormalities may be seen. Here a band of white fibrous tissue arises from the disc and passes out to the periphery. These eyes are usually virtually blind.

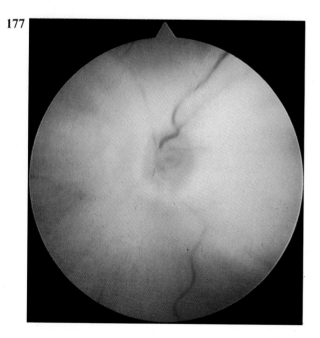

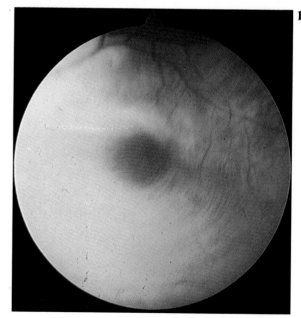

177 and 178 Rarely, large areas of myelinated nerve fibres may give the impression of a white pupil. The other eye was normal.

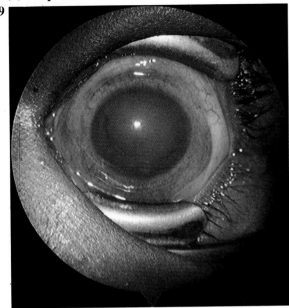

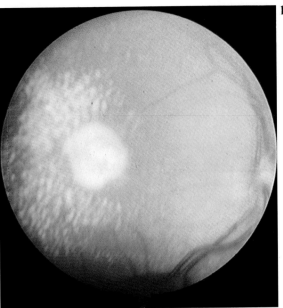

179 Buphthalmos may be confused with second-ary glaucoma seen with an advanced retino-blastoma (seen here). Closer examination will reveal the presence of virtually no anterior chamber with the lens-iris diaphragm pushed for-wards by a large white retrolental mass.

180 Coat's disease may appear superficially similar to a retinoblastoma but there are usually a considerable number of exudates present and, often, marked peripheral vascular changes with tortuous vessels and microaneurysms. Note the characteristic yellow colour contrasting with the pink hue of a typical retinoblastoma (Figure 150).

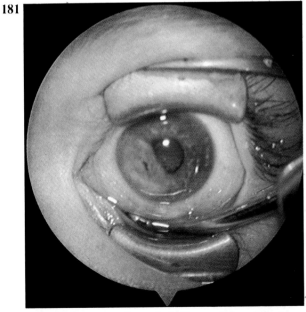

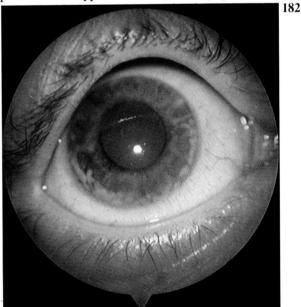

181 A naevoxanthoendothelioma; this can be con-fused with an iris recurrence of retinoblastoma (Figure 169) in which signs of pathology in the retina and vitreous would be obvious. Note the clear vitreous and normal red reflex seen here. Both these types of iris neoplasms can give recurrent hyphaemata.

182 An 'anterior uveitis'. Note the flocculent masses of cells. Aspiration showed the presence of retinoblastoma cells.

3 APPEARANCES AFTER CONSERVATIVE THERAPY

(a) Successful treatment

(i) Focal irradiation (e.g. cobalt plaque)

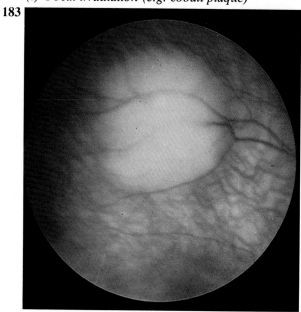

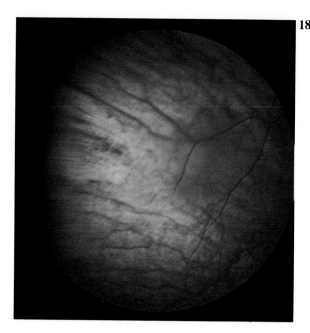

183 (Same case as Figure 184)   A classical medium-sized retinoblastoma ideally situated for the application of a cobalt plaque or other forms of focal beta or gamma radiation.

184   One year later shows the disappearance of the lesion and the scattered pigmentary changes consequent on the dose of radiation. These changes are localised to the site surrounding the base of the neoplasm. Note the small serous retinal detachment remaining.

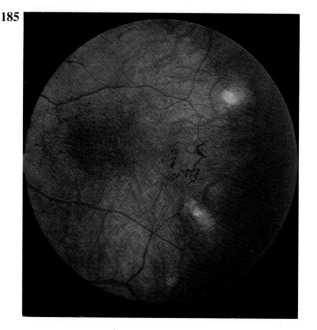

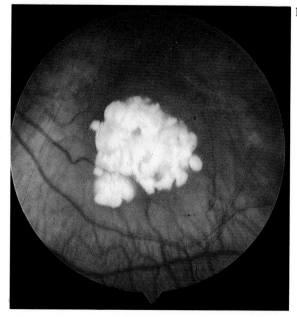

185   Occasionally after the application of focal radiation, there is complete disappearance of the tumour with slight pigmentary changes but neovascularisation appearing between the main retinal vessels.

186   At other times a calcified mass may occupy the site of the tumour, the area of calcification depending on the bulk of the tumour treated (see Figure 199).

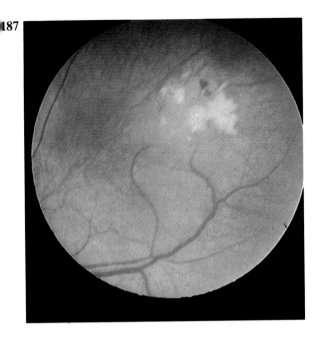

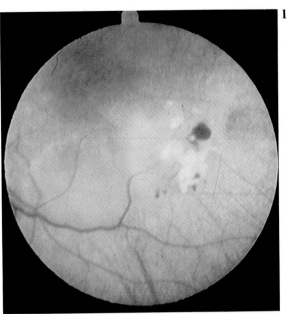

187 Sometimes regression of the tumour is composed of all the previous elements, *i.e.* serous retinal detachment, neovascularisation and calcification but these, however, do not remain static.

188 (Same case as Figure 187 – three months later) Note the increase in vascular changes and the slightly granular base because of early pigment clumping.

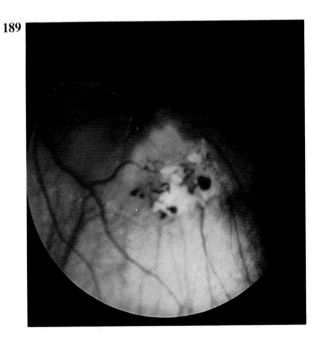

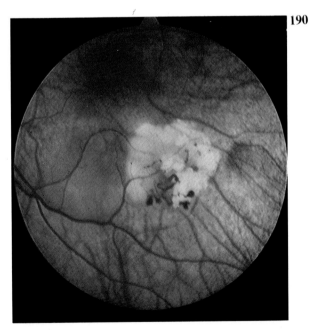

189 (Same case as Figure 188 – three months later) Further increase in the pigmentary and vascular changes and there is also a small rounded haemorrhage on the summit of the calcium. The serous retinal detachment is static but note the area of choroido-retinal atrophy around the base.

190 (Same case as Figure 189 – three months later) The haemorrhages have absorbed but the other vascular changes have remained static. The choroido-retinal atrophy is spreading.

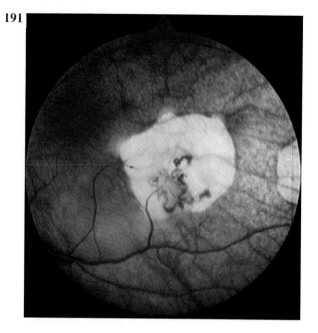

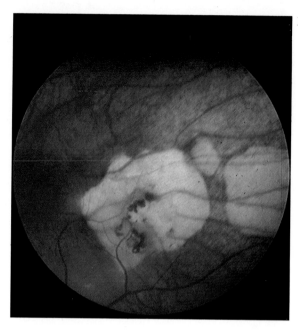

191 (Same case as Figure 190 – six months later) Note the marked increase in the neovascularisation, the obvious choroido-retinal atrophy around the base, together with the appearance of another small patch of atrophy.

192 (Same case as Figure 191 – one year later) Note the virtual confluence of the two patches of choroido-retinal atrophy and the disappearance of most of the choroidal vessels with marked surrounding pigmentary changes.

193 and 194 These photographs show similar changes after the treatment of a larger retinoblastoma nearer the disc.

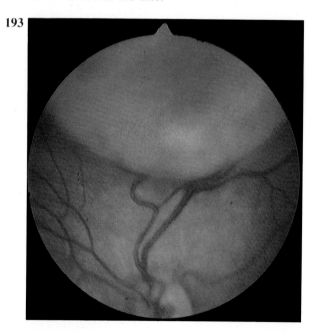

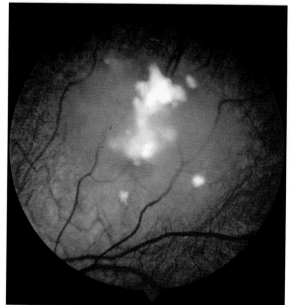

195 (Same case as Figure 194)   As larger vessels were involved a dense vitreous haemorrhage occurred later.

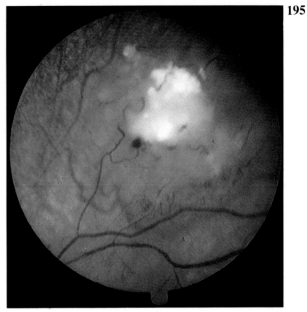

(ii) Whole-eye irradiation

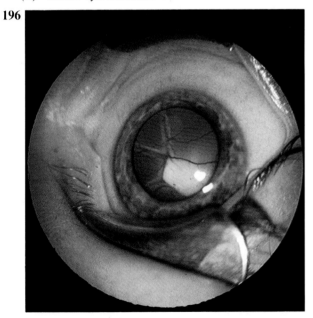

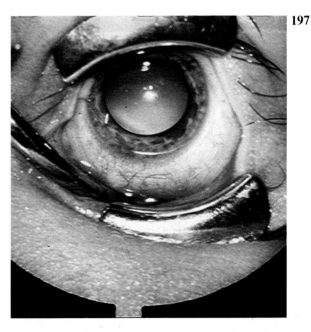

196   Shows a total retinal detachment caused by a 'sub-retinal' retinoblastoma.

197 (Same case as Figure 196)   After whole-eye irradiation the retina became flat with satisfactory regression of the tumour.

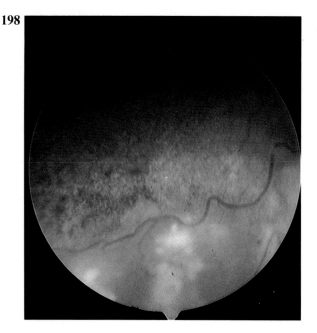

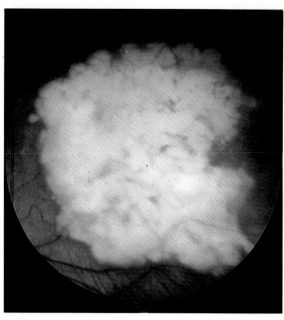

198 A retina that had become detached had reposited itself after treatment and the area is characterised by coarse pigment clumping, as seen above.

199 At other times large areas of calcium may become apparent at the site of the treated tumour.

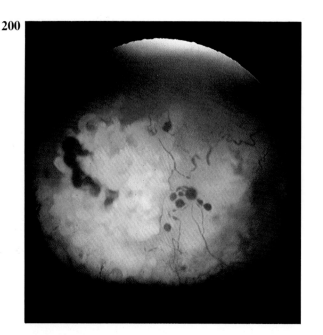

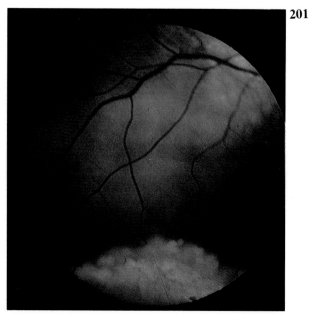

200 Occasionally, some large raised masses of calcium may contain telangiectatic blood vessels but these do not indicate malignant activity.

201 Less often, the large raised calcareous masses may be covered by a serous detachment which remains permanently. In this case, the inert debris is below a detachment, the only flat portion of the retina being that in the extreme upper part of the photograph.

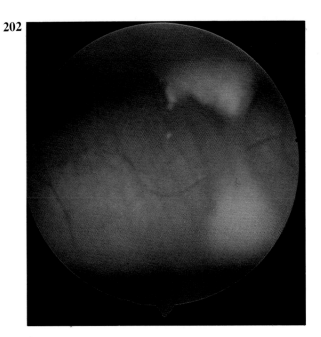

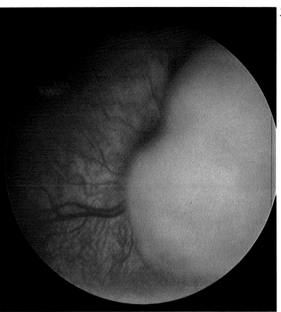

202 Rarely the detachment may be localised and become fibrotic. In this photograph the lower end of a large calcareous lesion (seen superiorly) is attached to a localised fibrous detachment leading to the retinal periphery.

203 Some retinoblastomata are not sessile on the retinal surface but pedunculated, as seen here. The optic nerve is hidden from view by the bulk of the tumour. Note the retinal vessels are normal indicating that the nerve was not involved by the growth.

(iii) Light-coagulation

A very useful therapeutic approach for small posterior tumours.

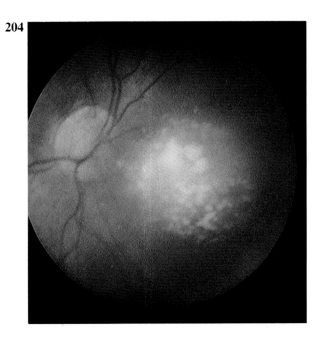

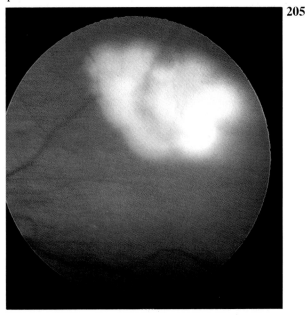

204 (Same case as Figure 203) Whole-eye irradiation (in this case by a Cobalt Beam Unit) produced regression of the tumour to inert debris adjacent to the disc.

205 Shows a tumour immediately after treatment. The pinkish tumour surface has been coagulated to a white oedematous mass.

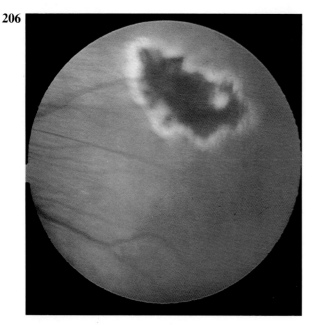

206 (Same case as Figure 205) The tumour has been eradicated. Note the heavy, even pigmentation induced by the light-coagulation.

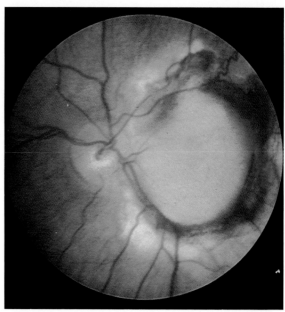

207 Large posterior tumours may need several courses of light-coagulation. Note the pinkish vascular tumour surrounded by a zone of pigment from previous light-coagulation.

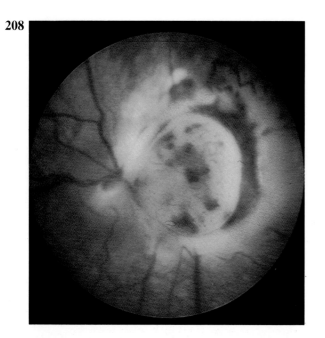

208 (Same case as Figure 207) Heavy light treatment has coagulated the surface of the tumour and ruptured some of the tumour blood vessels.

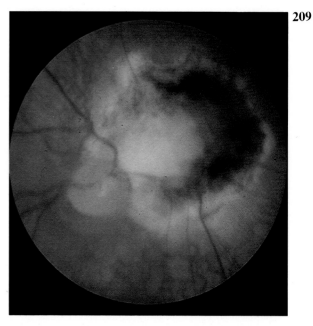

209 (Same case as Figures 207 and 208) The final end result. Note this tumour was situated on the nasal side of the disc. Such therapy would never be undertaken on the temporal side because of involvement of the papillo-macular bundle.

(iv) Cryotherapy

This type of therapy is very useful for the treatment of small anterior tumours.

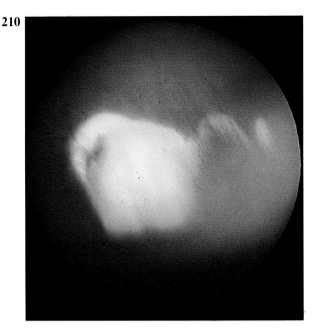

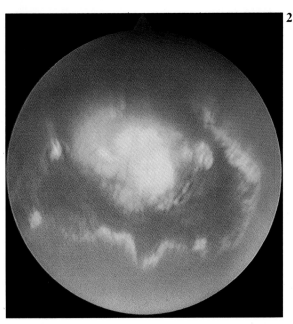

210   There is a small recurrence in an area of previous cryotherapy.

211 (Same case as Figure 210)   Further cryo applications were made with satisfactory regression. Note the pigment changes are more stippled and less dense than those following light-coagulation (Figure 206).

(b) Complications

These vary considerably from minor (which are merely extensions of some of the side-effects listed above) to major (which nowadays should be seen rarely). They will be dealt with on an anatomical basis.

(i) Lids and conjunctiva

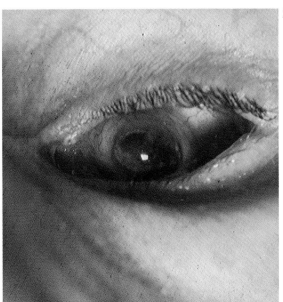

212   The end result of using too many focal types of gamma radiation (in this case, multiple radium applications used many years ago). The eye is shrunken and useless.

213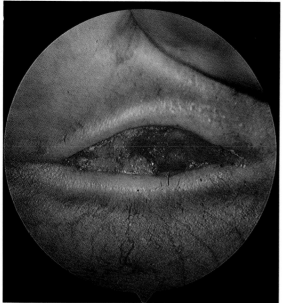

214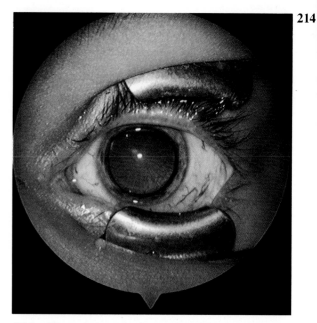

213 Occasionally, the orbit may have to be irradiated as a life-saving procedure in cases of extra-scleral extension of the tumour. The conjunctival sac invariably shrinks over the years as in this case, giving complete obliteration of the fornices. A facial prosthesis is the best way of dealing with this type of socket.

214 The conjunctival vessels often become telangiectatic to a minor degree either after whole-eye irradiation or after focal irradiation. Note the radiation cataract (see also Figure 222).

(ii) Cornea

215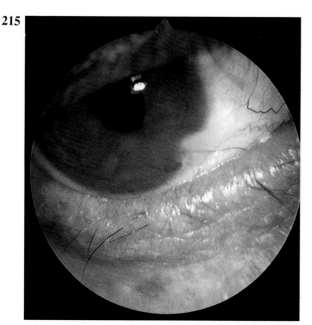

216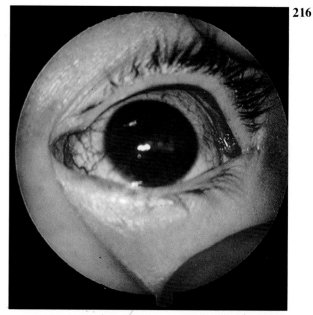

215 High doses of radiation (in this case a radon seed many years ago) may produce not only telangiectasia of the conjunctiva but also corneal changes. Here there is a 'pseudo-pterygium' leading to an area of localised corneal dystrophy (note the aphakia).

216 Occasionally, after heavy orbital irradiation the lacrimal gland becomes atrophic giving a 'dry eye'. In this case, atrophy of the orbital tissues has induced an exposure element giving marked corneal changes needing a tarsorrhaphy later.

(iii) Iris

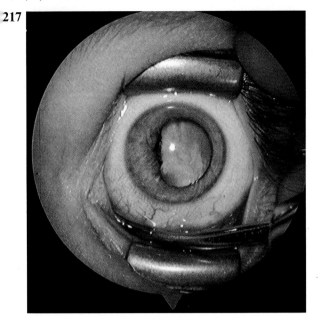

217 Irradiation of the whole eye may induce a low-grade iridocyclitis after other types of therapy. Note the broad-based anterior synechiae.

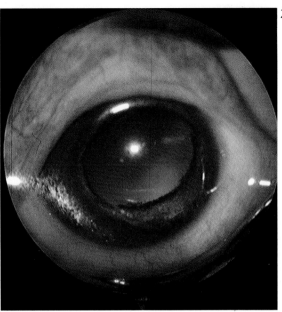

218 Focal irradiation techniques may induce segmental patches of iris atrophy.

(iv) Lens

Radiation cataracts may occur with focal irradiation techniques and always with external irradiation utilising a direct anterior field, but they are not necessarily progressive.

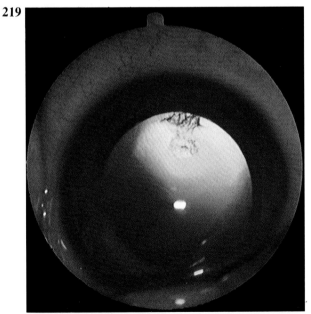

219 Shows a few globules in the lens adjacent to an area which received treatment with a cobalt plaque for peripheral retinoblastoma. These lesions are non-progressive and do not interfere with vision.

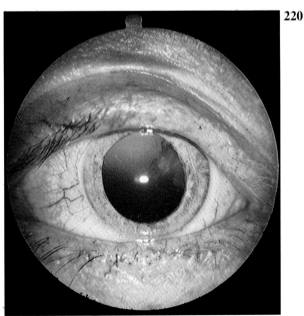

220 Shows a denser sectoral opacity following the application of a larger source of focal radiation.

221

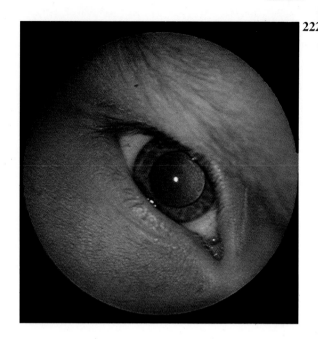

221 The earliest posterior sub-capsular axial globules characteristic of whole-eye irradiation. They may not progress.

222

222 The whole of the posterior cortex has become stippled with minute globules. This type invariably progresses.

(v) Retina

223

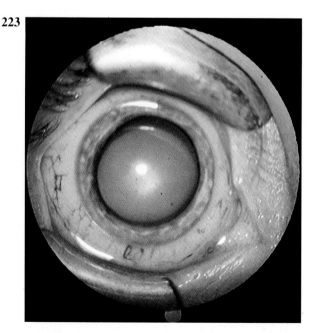

223 A typical dense white radiation cataract which is easily treated by aspiration.

224

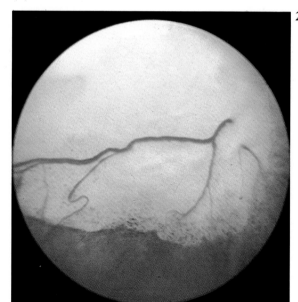

224 A severe form of radiation retinopathy following the application of a highly active form of focal radiation many years ago. This severe type of retinopathy should not be seen nowadays.

Index

Index

References are to page numbers